LIFE
AFTER
BABY

LIFE AFTER BABY

Rediscovering and Reclaiming
Your Healthy Pizzazz

Victoria Dolby Toews, M.P.H.

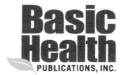

Basic Health
PUBLICATIONS, INC.

The information contained in this book is based upon the research and personal and professional experiences of the author. It is not intended as a substitute for consulting with your physician or other healthcare provider. Any attempt to diagnose and treat an illness should be done under the direction of a healthcare professional.

The publisher does not advocate the use of any particular healthcare protocol but believes the information in this book should be available to the public. The publisher and author are not responsible for any adverse effects or consequences resulting from the use of the suggestions, preparations, or procedures discussed in this book. Should the reader have any questions concerning the appropriateness of any procedures or preparation mentioned, the author and the publisher strongly suggest consulting a professional healthcare advisor.

Basic Health Publications, Inc.
28812 Top of the World Drive
Laguna Beach, CA 92651
949-715-7327 • www.basichealthpub.com

Library of Congress Cataloging-in-Publication Data is available from the Library of Congress.

ISBN-13: 978-15912025-8-5

Editor: Diana Drew
Interior design: Gary A. Rosenberg • www.thebookcouple.com
Cover design: Mike Stromberg

Printed in the United States of America

10   9   8   7   6   5   4   3   2   1

Contents

To my son, Dolby,
and my daughter, Sabine,
with love and appreciation.
You both gave me profound joy
in becoming a mother.

Acknowledgments

Working from a home office while raising children can be challenging at times. A special thank-you to my husband, Jeff, who didn't mind my ducking out of one more round of "balloon tag" or "aliens from the planet kushy-wushy" because I needed to finish something up in the office (some of the times I really did need to; other times—as he suspected and I am now publicly copping to—I just couldn't face one more round of balloon tag!). So thanks for not calling me on that, Jeff, and for every other way that you make my life wonderful!

With grateful appreciation, I thank all the new (and not-so-new) moms who shared their experiences and stories with me.

Introduction

From the moment your pregnancy test showed that you were pregnant, your body was no longer just your own. From then on, your thoughts likely centered on how you could make the best choices for the life growing inside you. Then, when your baby was born, you were probably too sleep-deprived and overwhelmed with the responsibilities of caring for a newborn to spend much time on yourself. Not surprisingly, you took a back seat to your new baby.

This is how it should be . . . at the beginning. But at some point it is okay to put yourself back on the list of priorities. For certain moms who are lucky enough to have a mellow baby who sleeps through the night early on, this could come after just a few months. But for the rest of us, it will definitely happen sometime within the first few years. Your body will never be quite the same as prebaby, but you can get to a new normal—and for some women this is an even healthier place than before they had a kid.

If you've picked up this book (or perhaps a well-meaning friend passed it along to you—nudge, nudge), then you're ready to devote a little more time to yourself. Consider this your road map to redefining yourself postkid.

Forget about the new-mom celebrities who look red carpet–ready mere weeks after childbirth. They have trainers, personal chefs, night nannies, stylists, and who knows what else. This is the real world, where new moms find that, on more days than they'd like to admit, pulling their hair back with a scrunchie takes the place of a daily shower.

This is not a book just about how to shed postbaby flab (although that will be covered in Chapter 1, "Losing the Baby Weight"); it's much more than that. It's about everything a new parent is adjusting to—body and soul—based on sane, sensible, and realistic advice.

Starting a family may derail a mom's good food choices for herself. While you may be ensuring that your toddler gets nutrient-dense foods, you probably end up grabbing convenience and comfort foods for yourself. In Chapter 2, "Kitchen Table Woes," you will find out about sugar alternatives, the importance of fiber, how to sleuth out potential food sensitivities, and how to tell if you would benefit from digestive enzymes. In Chapter 3, "Supercharge Your Nutrition," you'll learn even more about some key foods that can really crank up the nutritional quality of your diet, as well as the lowdown on organics and why antioxidants are so important.

As a nutritional backup plan, consider taking a daily multivitamin/mineral supplement, as explained in Chapter 4, "Supplement Savvy." You'll learn which nutrients most often fall short in a woman's diet, when is the best time to take your supplements, what are safe amounts to take of the most common vitamins and minerals, why women on the pill need to give special attention to their supplement plan, and get answers to your questions about kids and supplements.

Exercise is the key part of a weight loss plan, as you'll learn in Chapter 5, "Fitting in Exercise." Find out how to design a new exercise plan, protect yourself from sports injuries, and the best nutritional support for athletic moms.

From postpregnancy acne to stretch marks, having a baby can wreak havoc on your looks. Turn to Chapter 6, "Rediscovering Beauty Basics," for detailed information and tips about caring for your skin, hair, nails, and teeth.

And what about your sex life? You can find ways to balance your intimate relationship with your new role as a mom in Chapter 7, "Reconnecting with Passion." Learn here about why your libido seems to be on hiatus and natural ways you can lure it back.

The topics of getting enough sleep and staying awake when sleep isn't an option are biggies for new parents. Check out Chapter 8, "Fighting Fatigue," if you are looking for ways to nutritionally bolster your energy levels, as well as information about treating insomnia, chronic fatigue syndrome, and restless leg syndrome.

It's normal to feel thrilled to be a new mother, but it's also okay to feel other ways at times: frustrated, scared, overwhelmed, and confused. You'll find ways to cope with those feelings in Chapter 9, "Stress and Sanity."

As soon as a woman gives birth, it sometimes seems as if there isn't any more discussion about or attention paid to the mom (well, aside from postpartum depression). But there is so much going on with a new mom's body and mind in the year (and longer) after birth. Many women find that their own health is shunted aside in place of family and job demands, yet there are many health concerns that are unique to this period. You can find information and natural remedies for these health troubles in Chapter 10, "After-Baby Health Concerns."

Detailed safety information about every single herb and supplement mentioned in this book appears in the Appendix, "Herb and Dietary Supplement Safety." However, keep in mind that even if certain herbs or supplements have been safely used for many years, there is often a lack of scientific data specifically relating to pregnant and lactating women. Consequently, the safety picture with herbs and supplements is far from complete for these demographics. When the information is available, you'll see specific warnings about and contraindications involved with some of the herbs and supplements discussed in this book. But it is also important to keep in mind that pregnant or breast-feeding women should not use any medication or dietary supplement without their health care provider's input. And readers with specific health concerns should work with their doctors to ensure that a particular supplement does not interfere with other conditions or treatments.

CHAPTER 1

Losing the Baby Weight

Of course you've gained some weight; you've just grown a human being from scratch, for goodness sake! But now that the new person has vacated the premises, you're probably ready to get your old body back. Although it may not feel like it right now, good health and a slimmer waistline are within reach.

It's important to be patient with yourself and not try any drastic weight loss schemes. At a couple of weeks' postpartum, it's normal to still look five months' pregnant. In fact, it's helpful to think of pregnancy as an eighteen-month journey: It takes nine months to gain weight during pregnancy and at least another nine months postpartum to return to a prepregnancy shape. You might feel anxious to drop the extra pounds, but now is not the right time for an extreme diet, especially if you're breast-feeding. Nursing moms need to continue eating enough calories to support lactation.

"I was so ready to drop the baby weight that I was skipping meals sometimes, but when I realized that my milk supply was being affected, I knew that I couldn't rush the weight loss when it meant my new daughter could suffer," shares Liz. "Instead I focused on getting outside and walking with my baby while making healthy food choices, and the weight did slowly—ever so slowly!—come off."

WHAT'S A REALISTIC WEIGHT LOSS GOAL?

For years, nutritionists and weight loss experts believed that weight management was a simple equation of calories in versus calories out; that is, what you ate compared to exercise. To be blunt, losing weight hinged on willpower. Today, researchers are discovering that body weight is a much more complex equation, involving physical, psychological, social, and even genetic factors.

By the same token, just because your parents are overweight doesn't mean you should resign yourself to a lifetime of being heavy. You *can* lose weight and keep it off. The key is setting realistic goals. Remember, it took a long time to gain the weight; it's not going to come off overnight.

Gradual weight loss, no more than two pounds (0.9kg) per week, is your best bet for permanent weight loss. To determine how many weeks it will take to reach your ideal weight, simply divide the number of pounds you want to lose by two. For example, if you are 142 pounds (64kg) and want to be 130 pounds (59kg), you will need at least six weeks to meet your twelve-pound (5kg) weight loss goal.

Keep in mind that long-term weight loss is more likely when weight is lost in small increments (no more than ten to sixteen pounds [4.5–7kg] at a time) and the new weight is maintained for at least six months before attempting further weight loss. And don't forget that the changes you make to reach this goal need to be ones you can live with for the rest of your life.

THE METABOLISM—WEIGHT LOSS CONNECTION

Your body requires a certain amount of energy from food in order to keep functioning; this is called the basal metabolic rate (BMR). The BMR is the energy expended in the basic functions of breathing, pumping blood through the body, and maintaining body temperature. Not everyone requires the same amount of energy to sustain BMR; it's shaped by many factors, such as genetics, food choices, and even exercise.

Just as different automobiles get different mileage, depending on their fuel efficiency, people also have various "food efficiencies." Very efficient body types may be able to "travel" a long distance on modest amounts of food, with plenty left over to store in fat reserves. Our cave-dwelling ancestors no doubt appreciated this food efficiency, but in today's modern times with ample food supplies, the ability to pack on the fat is anything but an asset.

Virtually every dieter trying to slim down has resorted to restriction diets that involve either slashing calories at each meal or skipping meals entirely. But much to a dieter's dismay, this dieting technique actually encourages rebound weight gain. Weight loss experts now understand that limiting food intake works against weight loss goals by slowing down a person's metabolism.

Once metabolism is impaired, weight will be gained back faster than ever before—even when fewer calories are consumed. This is the yo-yo effect. The key to long-term weight loss is a "revved-up" metabolism that burns up calories, rather than a sluggish one that greedily stores calories as fat. Exercise is one healthy way to supercharge your metabolism.

HOW IMPORTANT IS EXERCISE?

The role of exercise in health is covered much more extensively in Chapter 5, but it's well known that exercise is an essential component in healthy weight management.

Skipping meals and surviving on fewer calories than the typical supermodel may result in short-term weight loss; but it's not healthy for your body, and you're overwhelmingly likely to gain back the weight (plus a few extra pounds) when you go off this unsustainable "diet." Admittedly, it lacks the sizzle of the latest best-selling diet book, but the "secret" of people who are successful at losing weight and keeping it off is healthy diet choices and lots of physical activity.

Numerous studies have documented that regular physical activity is one of the leading factors in whether a person trims down and stays that way. In fact, there is evidence that you can lose weight through exercise alone, even if you make no dietary changes.

Buy a Pedometer

Toning up may be as simple as buying a pedometer (it'll only set you back $5–$10). You'd be surprised how quickly ten thousand steps add up: park farther away from the mall entrance, walk to the park, take a stroll at lunch, and take the stairs instead of the elevator.

Exercise helps control your weight by using up extra calories that would otherwise find their way to your waistline as fat. Research shows that exercise has a suppressing effect on how many calories are eaten after a workout, and preferences for higher-fat foods may even decrease as a result of exercise.

As a baseline for a healthy body, experts recommend thirty minutes of moderate-intensity aerobic activity most, if not all, days a week, plus anaerobic strength training and stretching. Aerobic exercise, which includes walking, biking, jogging, swimming, aerobic dance, and cross-country skiing, is very effective at increasing metabolism and expending calories.

Anaerobic exercises, such as weight lifting, builds muscle mass and also burns some calories in the process. Having more muscle mass can aid weight loss efforts, since muscle burns more calories than fat. This means that even when you are standing in line at the grocery store, you are using more calories than when you had less muscle mass. One of the only perks of being heavy is a lower risk of osteoporosis; once you slim down you lose this protection, but anaerobic exercise can provide a measure of bone protection.

EXERCISE FOR WEIGHT MAINTENANCE

Study after study has shown the same sad news: lots of people are able to drop a few pounds, but far fewer are able to keep that unwanted flab off for good. But there is a glimmer of hope: The people who keep their trim new bodies for the long haul share some traits in common.

In fact, studies show that only 5 percent of people are able to maintain their weight loss after six months. Far too many people lose weight the wrong way—with crash diets—and then once they meet their weight loss goals, they go back to their old way of eating and the pounds pile back on.

The National Weight Control Registry (NWCR) concurs that weight loss maintenance is a real challenge. NWCR is a research group that studies successful weight loss strategies. All the NWCR research is based on people who have lost at least thirty pounds (13.5kg) and kept it off for at least a year. In other words, these are the people who have beaten the weight loss odds and know how to keep it off—these are the people you should emulate.

NWCR participants started out like many of us: about half were overweight as children, about half have one overweight parent, and nearly all of them had tried and failed to lose weight at least once. What changed for these seemingly average people that allowed them to beat the odds? Three main factors were noted: a greater commitment than ever before, stricter dieting, and a greater role of exercise.

Long-Term Weight Loss Success Stories

Those who shared their weight loss maintenance success stories with the National Weight Control Registry (NWCR) may have traveled different paths to reach their weight loss goals, but there were many similar strategies they all used to keep the weight at bay. The majority of NWCR participants:

1. Eat a low-fat, high-carbohydrate diet.

2. Eat an average of five meals/snacks each day.

3. Eat a majority of meals at home (as opposed to eating out).

4. Avoid fried foods.

5. Weigh themselves daily or at least once a week.

6. Exercise for about one hour a day.

7. Include weight lifting in their exercise plan.

There is no doubt that engaging in exercise is an important component for successful weight loss and maintenance. In fact, fully 90 percent of NWCR's success stories changed both diet and exercise. Remember, strength training is just as important as cardio. Many women are afraid to use weights, but they shouldn't be. Strength training revs up your metabolism, which means that your body is burning more calories each and every day.

And here's a little good news for those who want keep their hard-won success: it does get easier with time. A study of 758 women and 173 men who had lost at least thirty pounds (13.5kg) found that less effort and attention was required to maintain their weight loss the longer ago their initial weight loss had been.[1]

WHAT ABOUT A DETOX CLEANSE?

Using a detox or "cleansing" diet to flush toxins out of your body comes with the nice perk of lightening the scale. Clearing out toxic crud is a key step to getting healthy, and once that happens your body will naturally slim down.

There's nothing new about detoxification. Our bodies do it every minute of every day—through the colon, liver, kidneys, lungs, lymph glands, and skin—to clear out toxins as mundane as carbon dioxide and as exotic as food additives, heavy metals, medications, and cigarette smoke. This age-old process, however, can't always keep up with the onslaughts of modern life. By following a detox diet, you give your body a chance to catch up with this essential housecleaning chore.

Most people are sorely in need of some serious detoxing. If you decide to give this a try, choose a time to start a detox plan when you're mostly home and not traveling, since the foods you'll be eating for a few weeks aren't overly restaurant-friendly. But don't delay waiting for a "perfect" window, since that may never come. At some point, you may need to just leap into the program.

Extra weight (as well as many other health problems) may be traced back to toxic overload. Toxic chemicals (in air, water, cosmetics, clothes, and plastics) tell our hormones to do things we don't want them to do, such as pack on the pounds. More fat means more places for toxins to hide, and more toxins send your metabolism out of kilter and set the stage for even more weight gain. Detoxing may stop this nasty cycle.

A water- or juice-only fast is one way to go (but never for a nursing mom!), but there are more gentle (and just as effective) ways to cleanse the body. Even the more gentle cleanses should not be tried until you have weaned your baby. A one-week detox cleanse gives your body a chance to "catch up" with the need for toxic housecleaning.

One-Week Detox Cleanse Plan

1. Replace one meal each day with vegetable soup, vegetable juice, or a fruit smoothie.

2. Get rid of all processed foods, including high-fructose corn syrup, hydrogenated oils, refined grains, and artificial sweeteners, preservatives, and colors.

Is Your Home Toxic?

Once you've cleaned out your gut with a detox method, you don't want to invite the toxins back in. So, in addition to eating a cleaner diet, consider the toxins in your home.

- Keep a shoe-free home (lead, pesticides, and other toxic contaminants are tracked in by footwear) by slipping off your shoes at the door as you enter your home.

- Use a water filter.

- Wash your hands before handling food.

- Ditch aluminum foil for cooking and reheating and use parchment paper instead.

- Lower your fridge to at least 40 degrees Fahrenheit (4°C) and your freezer to zero (−17°C) or lower (to keep food bacteria and parasites on the run).

- Grow indoor plants (spider plants are a great choice) to clean the air.

3. For the other two meals each day, include only organic, wholesome "real food" ingredients, such as fruits, vegetables, nuts, legumes, beans, whole grains, lean meats and seafood, and nonfat or low-fat dairy products.

4. Eat lightly at meals, which means only until you aren't hungry, not until you are "stuffed."

5. Drink 6–8 eight-ounce glasses of filtered water each day (if you are urinating every one to two hours, then you know you're drinking enough water).

6. At the end of this one-week detox, transition back into regular eating, but continue to limit your intake of processed foods.

SLIMMING FOODS AND DRINKS

Pour a bowl of bran flakes, slice up some whole-wheat bread, or even try a fiber supplement. No matter how you do it, adding fiber to your diet really may make a difference in your waistline. And since a fiber-rich diet is healthy anyway, why not give it a shot? But don't expect to be a size six overnight. At best, extra servings of fiber-rich foods or fiber supplements are just part of an overall diet plan based on healthy, low-fat foods and exercise.

Fiber works by simply crowding other, fattier foods out of your diet. In addition, fiber blocks the absorption of fat in the intestines and slows down the eating process—so your stomach has time to tell your brain that you're full. Be sure to drink extra water while boosting fiber intake to minimize the risk of gastrointestinal upset.

Fiber doesn't have to come from just foods, either. People who use fiber supplements (such as psyllium) lose about twice as much weight as people who are just cutting back on calories.

Green tea might help with weight control, in part because tea boosts the body's rate of burning calories. The modest bump-up of energy expenditure caused by tea doesn't make it a miracle weight loss drink, but it does give dieters an extra boost that may get them over a plateau or keep them motivated.

Green tea seems to make an exercise-based weight loss plan more successful. Researchers have found that those combining exercise and a daily beverage supplying 625 mg of catechins (the antioxidants found in green tea) for twelve weeks lost more belly fat than those in a control group, who were also exercising but didn't get the green tea.[2]

Part of the reason green tea promotes weight loss is accounted for by its caffeine content. Caffeine increases the body's basal metabolic rate. This is referred to as a thermogenic effect and may boost weight loss efforts by helping the body burn more calories during day-to-day life. The potential effect on weight loss is small, but significant. Remember, pouring a cup of green tea with breakfast isn't going to be a miracle weight loss aid—a healthy diet and exercise program simply can't be replaced.

If you're close to your weight loss goal, eating more grapefruit might help you in the home stretch. The grapefruit diet fad of decades ago is being resurrected, but this time it is done in a more healthful fashion and with some real research to back it up. A clinical trial at Scripps Clinic in San Diego found that eating half a grapefruit three times daily or taking whole grapefruit extract (one capsule three times a day) resulted in weight loss. Intriguingly, this weight loss occurred without any other changes in diet or exercise. This Scripps study involved one hundred overweight men and women who lost approximately three pounds (1.4kg) each over three months, compared to a placebo group who did not include grapefruit in any form in their diets. Researchers suspect that one way grapefruit extract lightens the scale is by decreasing insulin levels (insulin is a hormone that regulates fat metabolism).

Forget bland—dish up some spicy, fat-burning foods. Adding the right spice is rumored to lessen the number of calories stored as fat from a meal. In effect, a spicy burrito is less fattening than a plain one. Develop a taste for turmeric, cayenne, hot peppers, and ginger. Although much of the research is anecdotal, many spices are thermogenic boosters; that is, they crank up your metabolic rate so you burn more calories in day-to-day life. As with any natural slimming aid, you can't expect to slather a burrito with guacamole and sour cream and have it "not count" caloriewise, just because it's spicy. These spices work best with other dietary and lifestyle changes.

WEIGHT LOSS SUPPLEMENTS

Although there is no magic pill that will miraculously and effortlessly melt away the pounds (kg) and inches (cm), current research does suggest that some dietary supplements may enhance weight loss.

7-Keto

7-Keto, a substance related to the adrenal hormone DHEA, acts as a non-stimulant, thermogenic fat burner. An accumulating body of evidence indicates that 7-Keto results in greater weight loss, compared to a placebo, when taken in the amount of 100 mg twice daily. In one study, 7-Keto was shown to increase metabolic rate during a diet, which will result in greater calories burned by the body.[3]

Bitter orange

Bitter orange (*Citrus aurantium*) works by stimulating thermogenesis, as well as by suppressing appetite and increasing lean body mass. There are numerous human studies of bitter orange (using 975 mg of bitter orange per day) showing that this supplement increases resting metabolic rate, curbs appetite, and induces weight loss.[4]

Calcium

You already know that osteoporosis-resistant bones depend on getting enough calcium in your diet (that's 1,000 mg for an adult woman), but keeping your bones strong could help you stay slim, too. According to research published in the *Journal of the American College of Nutrition*, women who have higher calcium intakes also have a lower percentage of body fat.[5] The researchers at California State University, Northridge took a look at the body composition and three-day diet records of forty-nine women. Not only did the women with more calcium in their diet have less body fat, they also carried less fat around their middle.

Coleus forskohlii

Several studies have found that forskolin, an extract from *Coleus forskohlii* promotes favorable changes to body composition. These studies of overweight men and women—involving twelve-week randomized, double-blind, placebo-controlled designs—taking 50–100 mg two to three times per day showed marked improvements in lean body mass levels and reductions in body fat percentages, body weight, and body mass index.

Chitosan

The fiberlike extract from crustacean shells, called chitosan, reduces fat absorption. Research finds that people supplementing with 1,500 mg of chitosan three times a day lose more weight and fat mass than those who don't.[6] Do not use this supplement if you are pregnant.

Chromium

The mineral chromium plays a role in the metabolism of fat and carbohydrates, as well as influencing the action of insulin. Chromium picolinate and niacin-bound chromium, in the amount of 100–300 mcg per day, both have been studied for improving body composition, namely losing fat while preserving muscle.

Conjugated linoleic acid (CLA)

Conjugated linoleic acid (CLA) is a slightly altered form of the essential fatty acid linoleic acid. The word *conjugated* in this context merely refers to some double bonds that are present in the fatty acid. Hamburgers and milk shakes are not where you usually think to look for the latest health-promoting nutrient, but that's where you'll find CLA. Because CLA is formed in the gut of ruminant animals (that is, cows and sheep), most of the dietary sources of CLA are meat and dairy products.

To a certain extent, the jury remains out on—and even a little bit perplexed about—this supplement. On the one hand, there is a robust body of animal research that clearly documents CLA's ability to lessen body fat and boost muscle gains in numerous animal species. But the human research has been less consistent, with some studies confirming body composition changes, and others showing no effect with CLA.

Following on the heels of numerous animal studies documenting CLA's ability to enhance fat loss and increase lean body mass, several human studies have been conducted. Half of the human studies (four of the eight) found small but significant reductions in body fat after supplementation with CLA.[7] For example, in one of the studies, overweight adults took either CLA or a placebo for twelve weeks.[8] Those taking CLA in the amount of 3,400 mg daily lost more fat mass.

Although there are few side effects reported by those taking CLA (a few isolated reports of GI upset), this supplement is not appropriate for everyone. Breast-feeding moms shouldn't use CLA because it has been shown to lower the fat content of breast milk; since babies need plenty of calories and fat in their diet, this could result in your baby not gaining as much weight as he or she should.[9]

HCA

The compound HCA, isolated from *Garcinia cambogia* and *Garcinia indica* fruits, blocks fat storage and serves as an appetite suppressant. Animal studies show that HCA slows the enzyme process that converts food into fat and suppresses appetite by sending signals to the brain that you've eaten enough (even if the meal was small). A large and growing body of research demonstrates that this supplement does enhance the weight loss process. For example, a placebo-controlled clinical trial showed that taking HCA resulted in greater weight loss in obese women taking 2,400 mg of HCA for two months.[10] Do not take HCA while you're pregnant or nursing.

Hoodia

Hoodia, also known as Kalahari cactus (although it is technically a succulent and not a cactus), grows in southern Africa where San Bushmen of the Kalahari have long used it to lessen hunger and thirst during long hunts. This traditional use of hoodia tipped off modern researchers to the potential of using hoodia for losing weight without feeling hungry.

Although the interest and hope for hoodia supplements seems to be outstripping the slow, plodding pace of scientific research, inroads have been made into the study of this bitter-tasting plant. Currently, there is not enough research to definitively establish hoodia as a weight loss tool, but researchers are beginning to determine how—and how well—this herb works to put a dent in how much food someone eats in a day.

A compound called P57 is the active ingredient in hoodia. There is only one clinical trial using human volunteers, and, unfortunately, its results have not been published. During the fifteen-day trial, nine adults took pills containing an unspecified amount of P57 extracted from hoodia twice a day. Compared to another group of nine adults taking placebos, the P57 group ate approximately 1,000 fewer calories and lost more body fat. Again, this study has yet to be submitted to the peer-review process and published in a scientific journal.

L-carnitine

Long-chain fatty acids are the primary source of energy in the human body, and one of the most important things that L-carnitine does is to transport these long-chain fatty acids into the mitochondria, where they are used to create energy. L-carnitine might be helpful for weight control through this association with fat metabolism. Research with overweight people supplementing with 1 gram of L-carnitine daily for three months (while also making changes in diet and exercise) reported greater weight loss. However, other research has not found a beneficial effect of L-carnitine on weight loss.

Licorice flavonoid oil

Licorice flavonoid oil has been found in a double-blind clinical trial of 103 overweight individuals to reduce body fat mass over a twelve-week period of supplementation with 300 mg per day.[11] Licorice should not be taken during pregnancy.

Multivitamin/mineral

Unfortunately, many women dieters eat less than the ideal diet in their weight loss efforts. National surveys have found that dieters frequently eliminate entire food groups while they diet. This places many dieters at risk for vitamin and mineral deficiencies. Consequently, a vitamin and mineral supplement may never be more important for a woman than when she is dieting.

Pyruvate

Pyruvate is a compound formed in the body as carbohydrates and protein are converted into energy. Several foods, including red apples, cheese, dark beer, and red wine, contain small amounts of pyruvate. Scientists suspect that pyruvate enhances the use of fat as a source of energy and cranks up metabolic rate. In any event, the end result is well documented in clinical trials: pyruvate, in the amount of six grams daily, leads to greater weight loss.[12]

Vitamin D

The more vitamin D circulating in your bloodstream, the lower your body weight tends to be.[13] On average, women lacking in this sunshine vitamin are heavier by more than sixteen pounds (7kg) when compared to women with adequate levels of vitamin D. Women with a vitamin D shortfall also rank 3.4 points higher in body mass measurements. Considering that more than 60 percent of young women don't get enough vitamin D (even women who live in sunny California, as in the study finding this vitamin D deficit), it makes sense to supplement with 800 mg vitamin D daily for a trimmer figure, as well as overall health.

White-bean extract

Double-blind clinical trials with white-bean extract, a starch blocker, find that overweight adults supplementing with 445 mg of this compound lose more weight and waist circumference, compared to those taking a placebo.[14]

Yerba maté

Yerba maté, a South American herb, lengthens the time it takes for the stomach to empty and leads to a quicker feeling of fullness. Clinical research shows that this supplement in the amount of 300 mg per day results in greater weight loss.[15] Do not use this herb during pregnancy or lactation.

WEIGHING IN

Remember, there's no substitute for a healthy, low-fat diet and regular exercise in the battle of the bulge. But you can give your body some extra support from Mother Nature. One of these antifat herbs, minerals, amino acids, or other natural supplements may give you just the edge you need to get over your "dieter's plateau." But the more important take-home message is this: a woman who is content with her body, despite a few extra pounds, is much more attractive overall than one who is obsessed with her weight.

CHAPTER 2

Kitchen Table Woes

Sure, you ate well during your pregnancy; you were providing nutrients to a growing baby, after all. But why does it matter what you eat now that the little one is out in the world? Healthy foods will help your body heal, keep your energy level up, and (if you're nursing) pass along the best nutrients to your baby.

"For me, having kids has both helped and hurt my nutrition choices," shares Mary Pat, a mom of two. "While I tend to have healthier foods in the house for my kids, on the other hand, I've been known to go the chocolate route when I am exhausted and stressed or haven't had a chance to eat right because I am too busy caring for my kids . . . and that happens a lot," she admits.

DON'T STOP EATING WELL WHEN THE BABY IS BORN

The time surrounding pregnancy, nursing, and having young children is a wonderful opportunity to rethink your eating habits and lifestyle. Smart choices pay off for both mom and baby and, if they become habits, may bring health benefits long after the baby is born.

Unfortunately, eating right is not an instinctive process, as evidenced by the Standard American Diet. The Standard American Diet really lives up to its acronym: SAD. Although there are signs of improvement recently, nutrition surveys repeatedly find that the drastic changes that occurred to the American diet over the past century have not been good overall. In fact, a step backward would be a positive change.

How the American diet evolved from the early 1900s until today mirrors the complex relationship among technology, economics, and social changes that have also occurred. Our grocery store shelves are now lined with foods with practically no expiration date, but chock-full of preservatives, stabilizers, artificial colors, flavor enhancers, and a host of other laboratory-derived additives. A far cry from fresh eggs gathered from the barn or fruit off a tree in the backyard. The nutritional quality of many foods in our grocery stores today bears little resemblance to that of the basic foodstuffs of yesteryear. A step backward to the diet of our great-grandfathers would be much healthier than the "new" and "improved" products that show up in boxes and plastic bags on grocery shelves today.

GOOD FOOD LINKED TO GOOD HEALTH

This entire chapter could be boiled down to a three-word sentence of advice: eat real foods. It's easy to know if your foods are good for you. Good foods go bad, while bad foods stay good on the shelf for a long time (think Twinkies).

People who eat generous amounts of fruits and vegetables (compared to those who eat such foods sparingly) have a reduced risk of many diseases such as stroke, type 2 diabetes, several types of cancer, heart disease, and high blood pressure.

Fruits and vegetables provide fiber, vitamins, minerals, and phytonutrients that account for these health perks. As such, the Centers for Disease Control and Prevention have set the goal of getting the majority of adults to eat at least two servings of fruit and three servings of vegetables (with at least one of these being dark green or orange) daily. Unfortunately, according to the latest data, less than one-third of adults currently achieve this goal for fruit and vegetable intake.

Nutrition surveys generally find that nearly six out of ten Americans don't eat a balanced diet on a regular basis, although people who take supplements fare slightly better, with 84 percent aiming for a wholesome diet. Even those who meet or exceed the fruit and veggie goals may find it tough to get optimal amounts of certain nutrients, such as essential fatty acids and a wide array of phytonutrients. This is where nutritional supplementation may help. In other words, eat the best you can and take supplements to fill in any gaps (more on that in Chapter 4).

WHY WATER'S IMPORTANT

Americans take in a shocking amount of empty calories from sweetened beverages. Switching to water as your main drink of choice is a simple change that can have wide-ranging benefits. For nursing moms, it's also good to know that drinking plenty of water boosts your milk supply (breast milk is 87 percent water, after all), and for anyone, water keeps the digestive tract moving along and even fills you up.

Fast Food Face-lift

With laundry and dishes piling up, a baby up half the night fussing, and work and family obligations left and right, there's good reason that most of us find ourselves grabbing a haphazard meal more often than usual after becoming a parent. But it is possible to eat out and still eat healthy.

- Choose foods that include vegetables, like a sandwich with veggies or a stir-fried dish.

- Buy a meal and share it; many fast-food servings can easily feed two.

- Drink water instead of soda.

- Try the kids' menu (if there's something healthy on it); most restaurants' kid-size servings are enough for adults.

- Don't be afraid to try something different, like a California spring roll (sushi with veggies) or a new healthy menu item.

Most people live their lives slightly dehydrated (which can make you feel cranky, fatigued, and less able to concentrate—just what new moms don't need!). This is even truer in the hot summer months. A baseline amount to aim for is 8 eight-ounce glasses of water every day; you'll need even more if you're nursing.

Having trouble drinking enough water every day? Stock your fridge with filtered or bottled water; research shows that people drink more water when it is cold, as opposed to room temperature.

Tired of plain water? Try green tea. Drinking several cups of green tea daily reduces your risk of heart disease, stroke, osteoporosis, cancer, and even dental cavities. Although green tea contains the most disease-fighting antioxidants, black tea and oolong tea also contain a good dose of these healthy compounds and may be consumed if you prefer their flavors. As a bonus, green tea also provides a stress-busting compound called L-theanine.

A SPOONFUL OF SUGAR

If you're like me, the stress and boredom of taking care of a baby might drive you to the comforts of sweet, sugary treats more often than you'd like to admit. But you've probably noticed that gorging on sugar doesn't leave you feeling that great in the long run.

There are ways to get a sweet treat without going overboard with sugar. Historically, choices have been limited for anyone who wanted to cut back on sugar, yet still indulge in sweets. Even today, sugar (sucrose) accounts for more than 90 percent of nutritive sweeteners (meaning the sweetener supplies calories) used worldwide. However, there are more options in sugar substitutes and alternative sweeteners available in the marketplace than ever before.

Nonsugar sweeteners started life with a shaky reputation, when saccharin (the first sugar substitute)—sold under the brand name Sweet 'N Low—was suspected of increasing the risk of bladder cancer. Although saccharin-containing products are no longer required to carry a warning label, many of us have understandable and lingering doubts about saccharin and are anxious to find new sugar alternatives. Currently, sucralose (brand name: Splenda) garners the largest market share, although aspartame (Equal and NutraSweet) and acesulfame K (Sunett) remain steady sellers as well.

Only some of the above-mentioned sugar substitutes can be used for cooking, since not all do well when exposed to heat. Also, sugar does more than impart a sweet taste in certain recipes; it sometimes contributes volume, moisture, and tenderness, or promotes browning. Recipes that don't call for any baking or rising are the easiest to adapt to sugar substitutes. One reason consumers gravitate toward Splenda is that it can be easily used to replace sugar for both cooking and baking. Splenda replaces sugar on a cup-for-cup basis, although recipes with Splenda do cook a bit more quickly.

Although Splenda, NutraSweet, and the other artificial sugars sweeten snacks and drinks with no or greatly reduced calories, using these artificial sugars doesn't actually help people lose weight, according to the latest and most comprehensive review of sugar substitutes. In short, this study casts serious doubts on the main reason many people use artificial sugars: to lose weight.[1]

Yet, at the same time, research finds that sweets are a major culprit in this country's obesity epidemic. The average person consumes an extra fifty calories each day of sweetened drinks (soda and coffee beverages) compared to twenty years ago.[2] This translates to five pounds (2.25 kg) of weight gain every single year. So if artificial sugars, such as saccharin are out, what's a health-conscious dieter to do? This is where newer sugar alternatives step into the story in a big way.

There are a growing number of nonwhite-sugar sweeteners now available; and these newcomers are made by Mother Nature, not in a laboratory. There's sure to be one to fit just about anyone's needs. Get to know some of the more popular ones, as well as a few up-and-coming sweeteners that will be on grocery shelves soon.

Agave: This nectar comes from the agave plant. It's sweeter than sugar, so less can be used. It doesn't cause as much blood sugar fluctuation as sugar.

Amasake: Fermented sweet brown rice is a traditional Japanese sweetener called amasake. It can be used in cooking or baking.

Barley malt: This thick liquid sweetener, made from sprouted barley, has a maltlike flavor; it contains enzymes and protein.

Brown rice syrup: This is made from sprouted brown rice.

Date sugar: A powder made from dried dates. Since it contains whole dates, it provides all the nutrients and fiber found in dates. It replaces sugar on a cup-for-cup basis and is especially good for replacing brown sugar.

Evaporated palm sugar: Rich in nutrients such as amino acids and B vitamins, it's made from the juice of coconut palm sugar blossoms that are boiled and then ground into a powder. It causes less blood sugar fluctuation than white sugar and can be used on a cup-for-cup basis in place of sugar in cooking.

Evaporated sugar cane juice: As its name implies, this is simply the solids that remain when sugar cane juice evaporates. It's considered less refined than white sugar.

Fruit juice concentrate: This sweetener is cooked-down fruit juices (generally peach, pineapple, grape, and pear); it's generally found frozen.

Honey: This sweet fluid, produced by bees and stored in the honeycomb, has been consumed as both food and medicine for thousands of years.

Maple syrup: This sweetener is made by boiling sap from maple trees. It can be used as a topping or for cooking.

Stevia: This intensely sweet herb contains zero calories and is 100–400 times sweeter than white sugar. It's available as a powder or a liquid extract. A little goes a long way; just one teaspoon (5 ml) can replace one cup (200 ml) of sugar. Appropriate for use in beverages, as well as for cooking (although it helps to add unsweetened applesauce since only a small amount of stevia is needed). This South American herb even has medicinal properties, such as lowering blood pressure.

Xylitol: About as sweet as sugar, but with far fewer calories, xylitol can be found in gums and candies, but is hard to find as a tabletop sweetener. As opposed to sugar, xylitol actually promotes healthier teeth.

Yacon: Yacon is a potatolike root vegetable from Peru. Yacon syrup is a sweetener extracted from the plant. It can easily be used in beverages or in place of molasses or maple syrup.

FABULOUS FIBER

There are two types of fiber—insoluble and soluble. The difference between them is simple: one absorbs water (soluble); the other does not (insoluble). Whole grains, wheat bran, nuts, and vegetables are good sources of insoluble fiber. Soluble fiber can be found in oats, oat bran, barley, legumes, psyllium, flax, apples, and citrus fruits. Both types of fiber are necessary and beneficial. The National Fiber Council recommends that women get 28 grams of fiber daily. In reality, most Americans don't reach even half of this recommendation (surveys indicate that adults, on average, consume a paltry 10–15 grams of fiber daily).

Chances are good that you could use a bit more fiber in your diet. When boosting your intake of fiber, it's important to increase it gradually, since a sudden surge in fiber intake could leave you feeling bloated and gassy. Give yourself a couple of weeks to transition from a low-fiber to a high-fiber diet. Easy ways to add more fiber include switching from white to whole-grain bread, snacking on nuts instead of chips, upping your intake of whole fruits and vegetables, or eating a bowl of oatmeal for breakfast.

Make sure you drink plenty of fluids (at least eight glasses of water a day) when switching to a high-fiber diet, since fiber absorbs water in your digestive tract, so that your stools are softer and easier to pass.

Reaching the recommended fiber intake doesn't mean just consuming fiber-rich foods. Many people might find it easier to rely on a fiber supplement, such as one based on psyllium, to boost their fiber intake. In addition to supplements based on psyllium, you can also find good fiber supplements made from flaxseed, fenugreek, and/or glucomannan.

When it comes to healthy bowel function, all roads lead to fiber. Fiber is key to bowel regularity, since it keeps everything moving along through the intestines. Both insoluble and soluble fibers are helpful in this regard. Insoluble fiber accelerates what's known as "transit time"; that is, how long it takes for food to go from start to finish in the digestive process. As an added bonus, insoluble fiber scours the intestinal walls with a mechanical sweeping action to remove old waste matter and toxins that could be stuck in the folds and crevices of the large intestine. While insoluble fiber adds bulk to stool, soluble fiber absorbs water to form a gel, which makes stool softer and easier to pass.

In addition to the "feeling better" perk of bowel regularity and resolving constipation and hemorrhoids, fiber has other important benefits for women, including protection against irritable bowel syndrome and breast cancer. As if that weren't enough, people who eat more fiber live longer. Clearly, there is everything to gain and nothing to lose by fitting in more fiber!

FINDING FIBER

FOOD	FIBER (GRAMS)
Lentils (1 cup [200 ml])	16
Black beans (1 cup [200 ml])	15
Instant oatmeal (1 packet)	6
Whole-wheat spaghetti (1 cup [200 ml])	6
Avocado ($1/_2$ piece)	5
Broccoli (1 cup [200 ml], cooked)	5
Apple (1 medium)	4

FOOD ALLERGIES AND SENSITIVITIES

Food allergies are less common than many people think. Only 2 percent of adults and up to 8 percent of children have a true food allergy, in which the body's immune system releases antibodies in response to a particular food. The end result of this allergic reaction may include anything from swelling in the mouth to stomach cramps, vomiting, diarrhea, hives, rashes, eczema, wheezing and other breathing problems, and, in the most dire cases, death. Cow's milk, eggs, wheat, tree nuts, peanuts, fish, shellfish, and soy top the list of food allergy culprits.

Food sensitivities are much more widespread than food allergies. With a food sensitivity (also called an intolerance) the problem doesn't lie with the immune system, but with the proper digestion of a food. For example, people with lactose intolerance may get cramps or diarrhea after drinking milk because they lack the enzyme lactase needed to digest milk sugar (lactose). Other common food intolerances include the inability to digest gluten in wheat (celiac disease) and sensitivities to food additives, preservatives, and artificial colors.

People with a true food allergy will need to avoid their trigger food(s). Although, over time, some people outgrow a food allergy to milk or eggs, especially if the food has been avoided for several months, allergies to nuts, fish, and shellfish have no cure and tend to last a lifetime. Taking the enzyme lactase when eating dairy products may treat lactose intolerance, but for the other food sensitivities, the problem food needs to be eliminated from the diet or only eaten in small amounts to avoid symptoms.

WHAT ABOUT DIGESTIVE ENZYMES?

Many people find that digestive enzymes improve their digestive process and resolve indigestion problems. This is particularly true for those who experience indigestion because the body no longer makes enough digestive enzymes. While there are medical tests to check on enzyme levels, it is often cheaper and easier to just give digestive enzyme supplements a try. If you experience bloating, gas, or excessive burping after a meal, digestive enzymes may be a helpful addition to your supplement regimen. Taking digestive enzymes during or after a meal is more effective than taking them before eating. Try 500 mg of bromelain, 25–50 mg of papaya enzyme, or, for pancreatic enzymes, follow the label directions.

Think of enzymes as the keys that unlock the nutrition of the food you eat. As people age, the body tends to make fewer digestive enzymes, so supplementing with digestive enzymes (either a single enzyme or a combination of enzymes) can replenish what the body needs for optimal digestion. A group of digestive enzymes known as "pancreatic enzymes" are commonly used as digestive aids; pancreatic enzymes contain a mix of enzymes that together help break down proteins, carbohydrates, and fats. Pancreatic enzymes literally come from the pancreas of animals (usually hogs).

The enzyme lactase digests lactose (milk sugar). Lactase enzyme supplements are particularly useful for those who are lactose-intolerant. Lactose-intolerant individuals do not make enough of this enzyme. When they consume dairy products, they end up with gas, cramps, diarrhea, and a generally upset tummy about thirty minutes to two hours after eating or drinking foods containing lactose. Most people's bodies make less lactase as they reach adulthood. About a quarter of Caucasian adults of northern European descent develop lactose intolerance, but 50–95 percent of people of other ethnic backgrounds become lactose-intolerant as adults.

Papaya enzymes serve as a natural digestive aid, helping to break down proteins. Papaya enzymes are a potent and tasty way to support the body's digestion, particularly during times of stress (when the body's own enzyme production might suffer). Papaya enzymes might be called "papain" on product labels. Papaya enzymes should not be used during pregnancy, due to a risk of uterine contractions. Bromelain enzyme comes from pineapple stem and fruit. It aids overall digestion, as well as being particularly adept at breaking down protein. Some people who prefer not to use pancreatic enzymes (given the animal source) use bromelain as a plant-based digestive aid substitute.

BPA AND HEALTHY KIDS

You've probably already heard about concerns with a chemical called bisphenol A (BPA). Seven billion pounds (32 million kg) of it is added to the world each year, much of it earmarked for food packaging. You can't pump this much of a chemical like BPA into the food supply and not expect it to trickle into the human body. And trickle it does. More than 90 percent of people (even including newborn babies) have BPA in their bodies.

Unfortunately, BPA doesn't stay put in food containers; it tends to leach into foods and drinks held within, and from there it gets into the human body and acts as an endocrine-disrupting chemical. Kids are particularly susceptible to BPA because their bodies are growing, their cells

Sleuthing BPA

If you're concerned about BPA exposure, here's a cheat sheet of products to avoid and which are a better bet.

Avoid These (unless the label says *BPA-free*)

Plastics (especially number 7)

Plastic baby bottles, teethers, and pacifiers

3- and 5-gallon (11-liter and 19-liter) water bottles

Canned foods and soups

Plastic cutlery

Dental sealants and composite fillings

Better Choices

Any product with *BPA-free* on the label

Glass, porcelain, or stainless-steel containers

Plastics (numbers 1, 2, 4, or 5)

Fresh or frozen vegetables

Cartons (such as Tetra Pak)

Dental sealants and composite fillings free from or low in BPA (your dentist can find out by checking the Material Safety Data Sheet for "BADGE," a chemical closely related to BPA, in the list of ingredients)

are dividing rapidly, and their organs are still developing. What's the big problem with endocrine disruptors like BPA? These nasty guys can change our genetic makeup, as well as meddle with reproduction, encourage the growth of fat cells, slow down metabolism, and tinker in a bad way with our brains. Alarming animal studies suggest that BPA might cause problems like early puberty, an increase in breast and prostate cancer, obesity, and attention problems.

Clearly, BPA is bad news. So what's a concerned family to do? For starters, choose BPA-free products for food preparation, serving, and storage, for baby bottles and water bottles for the whole family, as well as for objects that go in the mouth, such as pacifiers and teethers.

Since BPA tends to leach as plastics age, you'll definitely want to toss any bottles and cups that look worn or scratched and replace them with BPA-free items. Also, don't heat plastics or use them in or with boiling water, as BPA leaches even more with heat.

The U.S. Food and Drug Administration (FDA) has a plan to reduce BPA in the U.S. food supply, although no new regulations are yet in place. Manufacturers don't seem to be waiting. Numerous companies—especially those geared to babies and children—are already responding to long-simmering concerns about BPA by phasing out this chemical or offering alternative packaging. In the meantime, keep an eye on labels to select BPA-free products for your family.

CHAPTER 3

Supercharge Your Nutrition

Including nutritional superstars in your diet may help you get through the day during the high-pressure time of raising little ones. What you eat today is a key ingredient in how your body feels tomorrow. If you've ditched fast foods in favor of "real" foods, then you've already gone a long way toward helping your body run at its best.

Ready to go even further? Why not supercharge your diet with powerhouse "super" foods. "It's so true that I feel better when I start my day with yogurt and have a 'green' smoothie in the afternoon. It might sound corny, but eating superfoods does help me have a super day," says mom-of-three Erin.

NEW MOM SUPERFOODS

No doubt, as a mom, you're short on time and energy, so choose these quick, superfoods to get a good nutritional bang for the buck:

Chia

Chia is an edible seed with a nutty flavor that comes from a desert plant, and, yes, the same seed sprouts as "hair" on the novelty Chia Pets. Chia, which belongs to the mint family, is native to Central America, where chia seeds were a staple in the ancient Aztec diet. Chia is a particularly well-rounded food, providing protein, fiber, essential fatty acids (especially those coveted omega-3s), antioxidants, calcium, magnesium, manganese, copper, niacin, and zinc.

Unlike flax seeds, chia doesn't need to be ground before use. Use chia seeds in any recipe that calls for sesame or flax seeds, such as muffins, bread, or hot cereal, or sprinkle them on salads or yogurt. To make the drink called Chia Fresca, which is popular in Mexico and Central America, mix 1 teaspoon (5 ml) chia seeds with 1 cup (200 ml) of water and add lime juice and sugar to taste. Since chia does not go rancid as quickly as most other seeds, it can be stored at room temperature in a dry place for about two years.

Coconut oil

Coconut oil, derived from coconuts, contains a rare type of oil called medium-chain fatty acids. Coconut oil lowers the risk of heart disease, supports weight loss efforts, boosts immunity, and even appears to have cancer-fighting properties.[1]

There are two types of coconut oil: virgin and RBD (refined, bleached, and deodorized). Virgin coconut oil is less processed and more flavorful; however, many people prefer the RBD oil because it is colorless, tasteless, and odorless. Coconut oil doesn't need to be refrigerated and will stay fresh for several years. It is a great oil for frying.

Cruciferous vegetables

A diet rich in cruciferous vegetables (five or more weekly servings) offers tremendous health benefits. Cruciferous vegetables, including arugula, Brussels sprouts, broccoli, cauliflower, cabbage, and watercress, contain high levels of health-enhancing sulfur compounds as well as other important nutrients (vitamin C, folic acid, vitamin A, bioflavonoids, and fiber). Regular inclusion of these types of vegetables lowers the risk of cancer.

Fish

The omega-3 fatty acids in wild salmon help keep the heart healthy, which is why the American Heart Association recommends including two servings of oily fish (such as salmon, mackerel, or tuna) in your weekly diet. Salmon also provides plenty of protein, iron, and other essential minerals to the diet. If you're nursing or considering another pregnancy, fish is also very valuable because including fish on your weekly menu or taking a supplement of omega-3 fatty acids aids your baby's brain and retina development. For mom, omega-3s help prevent preterm delivery and depression during pregnancy.[2]

Flax

Flax seeds, which look like miniature apple seeds, are rich in omega-3 fatty acids and lignans. Flax has been linked to a lower risk of heart disease, depression, asthma, arthritis, and lupus. In addition, flax is a mild laxative.

Buy ground flax, or if you have whole flax seeds, grind them in a coffee grinder to improve digestibility. Store flaxseed in an airtight container in the refrigerator for up to two months. Add ground flaxseed to cereal, yogurt, salad, mustard, or include it when baking cookies, muffins, or bread.

Green foods

Green is the color of healthy plants, new growth, and healing. When it comes to green foods—the color green really lives up to its reputation. Although green foods come from a wide variety of plants grown on both land and water, what they have in common are seriously high nutrient levels squeezed into a ridiculously small space.

Green foods is a general term that refers to numerous chlorophyll-rich plants. The green foods category includes the micro-algaes spirulina, chlorella, and Klamath Lake blue-green algae; and cereal grasses, such as barley grass and wheat grass. Green foods are chock-full of antioxidants, vitamins, minerals, amino acids, and essential fatty acids.

Aside from their impressive nutritional profile, the other commonality with green foods is the magic stuff that actually makes them green: chlorophyll. The chemical structure of chlorophyll is almost identical to hemoglobin (the red, oxygen-transporting pigment in human blood), which is why chlorophyll is known as the lifeblood of the plant world.

And when we eat foods that contain chlorophyll, its powerful effects are available to our bodies; namely, potent antioxidant properties, the reduction of inflammation, and wound healing.

You can grow a small planter of cereal grasses and juice them (you will need a juicer that is robust enough to handle grasses); simply cut off a 2–3-inch (5–7.5-cm) round of the grass for each serving of juice. If you don't have the time, space, or inclination to do this, there are other ways to consume green foods. Green food powder or flakes can be mixed with water or juice. When mixing a drink, use 1–3 teaspoons (5–15 ml) of the powder or flakes, keeping in mind that the more you use, the stronger the flavor. Many people find the taste of these drinks to be quite strong; it might be more palatable to mask the flavor somewhat in a fruit or yogurt smoothie.

You can experiment with the different green foods to see if one tastes better to you, since they all have similar health effects. But what keeps people coming back to green foods is that you really can "feel" the benefits.

Hemp

Although hemp is in the same species as marijuana, hemp seeds (and the oil made from them) contain negligible amounts of the mind-altering THC substance. Hemp oil has a pleasant, nutty flavor. Hemp contains high levels of essential fatty acids, including both omega-3 and omega-6 fatty acids, vitamin E, and protein. Hemps seeds can be used as an effective bulk-forming laxative.

To try hemp, take 2–4 tablespoons (30–60 ml) of shelled hempseed or 1–2 tablespoons (15–30 ml) of hemp oil daily. For cooking, hemp seeds can be used in place of flax seeds in many recipes (such as muffins, hot cereal, or bread) and hemp oil can be used in place of other oils, in salad dressing, for instance.

Honey

Honey is the lovely, sweet substance that bees make from plant nectar. Honey is a delicious alternative to refined sugar and a source of antioxidants. Honey inhibits the growth of bacteria and promotes the healing process. Raw honey (which hasn't been pasteurized or filtered) is a great choice. Since honey is sweeter than sugar, to use it in place of sugar in recipes you'll only need one-half to three-quarters of a cup (100–150 ml) for each cup (200 ml) of sugar. Make sure to reduce the amount of liquid in the recipe by about one-quarter of a cup (50 ml). Foods with honey may brown more quickly than those made with sugar. Never give honey to a child younger than one year old.

Live-culture yogurt

As a quick snack, breakfast mainstay, or dessert ingredient, live-culture yogurt earns high marks for being an excellent source of protein, calcium, and health-promoting bacteria. The fermentation process used to make yogurt lessens the amount of lactose in yogurt (compared to milk), and many people with intolerance to milk can digest yogurt without any trouble. Including yogurt in your diet may improve digestion, immune function, and even boost the absorption of vitamins and minerals.

Mushrooms

Mushrooms offer a lot of good nutrition in a flavorful package. For example, the mushroom reishi has been used by Traditional Chinese Medicine as an "adaptogen," or general tonic, to promote overall wellness and vitality for at least the past three thousand years. Another mushroom, shiitake, has a strong enhancing effect on the immune system. Mushrooms are available in a variety of forms, including fresh, dried, powdered, tinctures, capsules/tablets, or tea. Consuming the whole, dried mushrooms (the "fruiting body") is the traditional way to use mushrooms. However, the other forms may sometimes be more convenient and are certainly viable choices. In fact, medicinal mushrooms are increasingly easy to find even in mainstream grocery stores and can be incorporated into any recipe calling for mushrooms.

Superfruits (Acai, Goji, Mangosteen, and Pomegranate)

Several highly nutritious fruits from around the world are more available than ever before, including acai berries from the Amazon, goji berries and mangosteen from Asia, and pomegranate from the Middle East.

All these superfruits contain impressive levels of antioxidants, and a diet including these fruits appears to strengthen immune function and lessen the risk of degenerative diseases, such as diabetes, arthritis, and cancer. Goji juice has an exotic taste, sweet and sour at the same time. Research shows that when healthy adults drink a goji supplement, they experience increased energy levels and a lessened stress load.[3]

Acai juice, which tastes similar to blueberry juice, is one of the best ways to try this superfruit, since fresh acai is not available in the United States (the berries don't last long enough to be shipped out of the tropical rain forest). Pomegranate juice has a sweetly tart flavor, which may be an acquired taste; eating the fresh fruit is another option.

Mangosteen juice tastes like a blend of strawberry and pear juice. Most mangosteen research involves the rind of the fruit (which doesn't make it into the juice), so if you want to try mangosteen for a specific health concern, use a product that includes the rind. All these super-fruits can be consumed daily or included in smoothies.

Sweet potatoes

The highly nutritious sweet potato has a thin skin and orange flesh. Sweet potatoes are naturally sweet and loaded with fiber, beta-carotene, vitamin C, vitamin B_6, and folic acid. They are a great alternative to plain potatoes.

ORGANIC FOODS AND THE DANGERS OF PESTICIDES

Organic foods are preferable and valuable for anyone, but the stakes are even higher for pregnant and nursing women, infants, and children. Exposure to pesticides may cause lifelong health complications.

Since young people eat more food (on a pound-for-pound basis) than adults, and tend to eat a less varied diet, the pesticide residues may accumulate quite quickly in their bodies. By choosing organics, you're going to be serving your child a meal in which the nutrients outweigh any chemical residue. The alternative is frightening, with research revealing that nearly three-quarters of the fruits and veggies eaten most often by kids have residues from pesticides—the average apple, for example, is contaminated with the residue from 3.2 different pesticides. Talk about some bad apples.

Children are particularly vulnerable to exposure to pesticides; in part, this is because they are less able to filter out harmful chemicals and because they are growing and developing rapidly. The potential pesticide-related harm to children is a laundry list of horrors for any parent: headache, fatigue, nausea, neurological disorders, lung damage, reproductive organ abnormalities, immune dysfunction, developmental problems of the endocrine system, birth defects, and cancer.[4,5]

Still wonder if all this talk about the dangers of pesticides is true? Well, wait until you hear about a study conducted by Elizabeth Guillette, PhD, a research scientist from the University of Florida. Dr. Guillette realized that she had a unique opportunity to compare the effects of pesticides in growing children.[6,7] Back in the 1950s in the Yaqui Valley of Mexico, the people living on the valley floor embraced the modern use of pesticides, while those in the foothills retained their traditional agricultural methods and avoided pesticide use.

Over a series of years, Dr. Guillette tracked the cognitive abilities of both communities. The differences in drawing ability of these children is striking and disturbing. There were profound differences in their ability to draw a person. The foothills children at ages four and five could draw a complete person. Among the pesticide-exposed valley children, most four-year-olds just scribbled, and the five-year-olds could draw a head and a line or a circle and a line. When researchers followed up with the children in the subsequent two years, they found that the seven-year-old exposed children were basically drawing on a four-year-old level. Meanwhile, the seven-year-old lesser-exposed children were identifying people by gender, with a dress or pants, appropriate hair, fingers, facial features, and shoes.

Can You Afford Organic?

After hearing about the pesticide perils of foods grown on a conventional farm, the question is no longer "Can you afford organics?" but

---

Saving Money on Organics

Expect to pay about 20 percent more for organic produce, but there are a few tricks to bringing the prices down. You might be able to shave a bit off your organic food bill by shopping smart, as noted below:

- Buy local products.

- Opt for in-season fruits and vegetables.

- Choose from grains and other foods in the bulk section of the grocery store.

"Can you afford not to serve them, when your child's health is at stake?" One out of every four Americans has decided that organics are worth it, and these people are already buying organic products.

Granted, organic food does cost more, but it certainly provides a better value. Organics are an investment in the future, and the prices are getting more competitive with conventional foods all the time. There are legitimate reasons that organic foods are more expensive, since organic practices include the more labor-intensive hand weeding of crops and organic foods are not subsidized to the same extent as conventional agriculture. In addition, many organic farms are still small and cannot take advantage of the economies of scale.

Many organic foods have gone head-to-head with their conventional counterparts, and researchers have found that the organics prevail. For example, corn and strawberries are packed with more antioxidant power when they are organic, and an extensive review of numerous food crops (including fruits, vegetables, and grains) found that the organics supplied significantly more vitamin C, iron, and magnesium than food grown using conventional agricultural practices.[8,9]

There is no question that young bodies absorb the pesticides from foods. Preschoolers in Seattle were divided into two groups, based on whether they ate organic or conventional foods. The levels of pesticides in their bodies were then compared.[10] For these two- to five-year-olds, the "conventional" group had much higher levels of pesticide metabolites in their urine than the "organic" group. In fact, the children eating a conventional diet had 8.5 times higher average levels than the children eating a mostly organic diet.

The bottom line from this study was that the simple change of consuming organic foods may reduce children's exposure levels from above to below EPA's chronic reference doses (how much of a chemical you can be exposed to on a daily basis throughout life before risking harm), thereby shifting exposure from a range of uncertain risk to a range of negligible risk. Consumption of organic produce represents a relatively simple means for parents to reduce their children's exposure to these harmful pesticides.

WHY FRUITS AND VEGETABLES ARE SO IMPORTANT

One of the reasons fruits and vegetables are so healthy for your body is that they are an excellent source of antioxidants. Antioxidants patrol the body, on the lookout for free radicals. Left unchecked, these harmful

---

Top Priorities for Organics

Pesticide residues are not in every food. For example, fruits and vegetables with thick skins, like citrus fruits and bananas, and nuts with shells, rarely have residues. The bad news is that some of kids' favorite foods, and the foods they need to be eating more of, may contain residues at levels of concern. It makes sense, then, to make these your top priorities for buying in organic form.

• Apples	• Juice	• Peppers
• Baby foods	• Lettuce	• Spinach
• Carrots	• Peaches	• Squash
• Grapes	• Pears	• Strawberries
• Green beans	• Peas	• Tomatoes

compounds damage the body and contribute to many diseases. Since free radicals influence the body at such a basic level, antioxidants are truly the first line of defense against degenerative diseases.

The body depends on many vitamins and minerals to act as antioxidants. The body is also equipped with antioxidant enzymes, such as superoxide dismutase, which neutralize free radicals. The best free radical protection comes from a diverse intake of antioxidants. Plant foods are an abundant source of antioxidant nutrients, such as vitamins A, C, and E, and the carotenoids. Antioxidants serve many purposes for the plants, including protecting plants from free radicals in their environment, such as those caused by ultraviolet radiation from sunlight. Fortunately for us, these benefits are transferred upon ingestion of the plant or plant extract.

ANTIOXIDANTS AND FREE RADICALS

Any discussion of antioxidants must include an explanation of what antioxidants are "against." Free radicals, or reactive oxygen species, are highly volatile molecules that are virtually unavoidable. Oxygen is a paradox. While oxygen is absolutely essential to life, too much of it is damaging to tissues and cells. It's analogous to electricity. Electrical wires are insulated to prevent injuries from the dangerous, but necessary, electricity within. Similarly, antioxidants "insulate" the body from the harmful effects of oxygen. It's a good thing antioxidants are around, because free radicals just can't be avoided.

Free radicals are formed from three primary sources: the body, the environment, and other free radicals. First, they are created within the body inadvertently during the complex process that generates energy from food. Exercise, illness, and certain medications may also increase the body's free radical load. The body, on occasion, even deliberately creates free radicals. As part of the immune system's response, invading bacteria and other infectious microorganisms are engulfed by specialized white blood cells. These immune system cells use free radicals derived from oxygen to kill the potential infection-causing agents. In this isolated instance, the body takes advantage of its enemy—free radicals—in order to stay healthy. Too often the reverse is true: free radicals are the instigators of ill health.

The second major source of free radicals is the environment. Toxins in the environment, either natural or human-made, are often free radicals. Air pollution, toxic waste, and pesticides introduce free radicals into the body. Ultraviolet radiation from the sun is another common environmental source of free radicals. Many times people introduce free radicals into their body through their behaviors. Each puff of cigarette smoke contains millions of free radicals; drinking alcohol also leads to the production of free radicals.

Thirdly, free radicals may be formed from other free radicals in uncontrolled chain reactions. Since a free radical molecule is missing a vital part of itself—one of its electrons—in an effort to restore the balance of a paired electron, it reacts with any nearby molecule in the body. What happens next is a deadly game of hot potato. As the original free radical "steals" an electron from another molecule, the second molecule becomes unbalanced. When an electron is taken from a molecule, oxidation is said to have taken place. The newly formed free radical then interacts with yet another molecule in pursuit of stability, and so on. These free radical chain reactions happen very quickly; in fractions of a second, but the end result may be devastating.

Free Radicals as a Source of Disease

Over time, free radical damage to the body leads to dozens of diseases and premature aging. For instance, free radical changes to LDL cholesterol are an early step in heart disease; DNA (our genetic blueprint) damaged by these reactive compounds may instigate cancer; and proteins in the skin mangled by free radicals may appear as wrinkles.

Antioxidants have the unique ability to donate the much-sought-after electron or remove the extra electron to stabilize free radicals. Antioxidants, therefore, stop the deadly chain of free radical reactions. This spent antioxidant is then either "recycled" by yet another antioxidant to avoid becoming a free radical itself or, if it stays in an altered state, its structure does not damage any other molecules.

The list of compounds that act as antioxidants is impressively long.

Besides vitamins A, C, and E, carotenoids, and selenium, the body pro-duces many enzymes that work to convert potentially deadly free rad-icals into harmless substances, such as water and ordinary oxygen. These enzymes include glutathione peroxidase, catalase, and superox-ide dismutase. In fact, it was the discovery of these antioxidant enzymes in the body that confirmed for scientists that free radicals could cause diseases and the body had developed ways to protect itself. These enzymes are found in every cell of the body; without them, we would literally spoil. In fact, antioxidant enzymes cease to function after death, which is the reason that tissues begin to rot.

Many things increase our free radical load, from stress to environ-mental toxins and a poor diet. Unfortunately, there is a limit to increases in the body's enzyme production; and we seem to have reached it as a society. Too often, it seems, the antioxidant defenses of the body are defeated and free radical damage accumulates and contributes to degen-erative diseases. Just as a general reinforces the army with new troops, our body's defenses benefit from reinforcements of antioxidant nutri-ents from the diet. Which is one reason why a nutritious and varied diet is so important to your overall health.

CHAPTER 4

Supplement Savvy

hances are, you aren't eating nearly as well as you think you are. Almost six out of ten Americans don't reach the goal of a well-balanced diet on a regular basis. And even those with stellar diets would find it tough to achieve optimal amounts of certain hard-to-get nutrients, such as vitamin D. This is why it makes sense to rely on a daily multivitamin/mineral supplement as a backup plan. Naturally, it's not an either/or situation; you'll still want to eat the best diet you can, while taking a supplement to fill in any gaps.

If you do decide to take a multi, don't get too worked up about which one you choose, since the best supplement regimen is the one you'll actually stick with. For instance, if your day is so hectic that you can barely find time to take a supplement once, let alone multiple times, then a one-a-day product makes the most sense for you. If you can, however, consistently take a multi two or three times a day, then by all means do that if you want, since multis designed for use several times a day offer more comprehensive benefits. The body can take better advantage of the complete span of nutrients when they come in smaller, divided doses.

DESIGNING A SUPPLEMENT PLAN

Start with a basic, no-frills multiple vitamin and mineral supplement. It's a simple, convenient, and cost-effective way to supply a balance of the most important nutrients. It may be a multi designed for adults in general or specific to women. A woman's multi differs from a man's multi in several crucial ways, with the main differences being more B vitamins and iron. There are four key nutrients for women that you should keep your eye on when setting up a supplement plan.

Folic acid

Folic acid is one of the essential water-soluble vitamins in the B-complex family (others in this family include vitamin B_6 and vitamin B_{12}). Folate is the form of this vitamin that occurs naturally in food. Even though it was one of the last vitamins to be discovered, folic acid is vital to almost every aspect of health.

All women of childbearing age, and especially all women who are pregnant, are urged to take at least 400 mcg of folic acid because it reduces the risk of a birth defect called neural tube defect. Too little folic acid in the first few weeks of pregnancy—often before a woman even knows she is pregnant—increases the risk of bearing a child with a neural tube defect (such as spina bifida or anencephaly), conditions where the embryonic neural tube that forms the future brain and spinal column fails to close properly. Supplementing with folic acid prevents up to 70 percent of these birth defects in a woman's unborn child.[1]

Need more incentive to reach for that bottle of folic acid every day? Recently, researchers from Spain found that four-year-olds whose mothers had taken folic acid stayed focused longer, had better verbal skills, and were more successful in social interactions than preschoolers whose moms didn't take this B vitamin during pregnancy.[2] Along a similar vein, Dutch researchers report that children of mothers who took folic acid supplements during pregnancy are at much lower risk of behavioral problems.[3]

Folic acid deficiency may play a role in some miscarriages. Women who had experienced several miscarriages were found to have lower blood levels of folic acid than other women.[4] The Dutch researchers who conducted this study advise folic acid supplementation for women having difficulty carrying a baby to term. Sound advice since folic acid is needed in so many ways for a healthy pregnancy.

Where to get your folic acid? The best dietary sources of this vitamin are dark-green leafy vegetables, brewer's yeast, orange juice, fortified cereals and grains, and broccoli. The U.S. flour supply began to be fortified with folic acid in 1998 (after which the incidence of neural tube defects decreased).

Folic acid is present in virtually all multivitamin/mineral supplements; it is also available as a stand-alone supplement or as part of a B-complex supplement. In a surprise twist, research shows that supplements of folic acid are actually a better way to boost blood levels of this vitamin than food sources.[5] All women should take 400 mcg of folic acid, but the recommended amount goes up to 800 mcg for pregnant women and 4,000 mcg per day for women with a history of pregnancy affected by a neural tube defect.

Calcium

Only one-quarter of American adults eat enough calcium-rich foods to meet the daily recommended intake for this mineral, which is 1,000 mg for adults. You know you need calcium for strong, osteoporosis-resistant bones, but getting plenty of this mineral also helps keep blood pressure in check, improves cholesterol numbers, makes preeclampsia in pregnancy less likely, and reduces the risk of colon cancer. As if that weren't enough of an incentive to pour a glass of skim milk, new research recently discovered that a woman's body fat goes down as her calcium intake goes up.[6]

Most people get the majority of their dietary calcium from dairy foods, but other potential calcium sources include tofu (check the label to make sure it was processed with calcium), calcium-enriched orange juice, sardines or salmon canned with bones, baked beans, almonds, kale, broccoli, and bok choy. Even with a healthy diet, you might want to consider a calcium supplement for extra insurance. This mineral takes up a lot of space in a multi, so you will probably need to take a separate calcium supplement to reach the recommended intake.

Get the most out of calcium supplements by taking each pill with a meal; you can only absorb a certain amount of calcium at a time, and food tends to improve calcium's absorption. There are many forms of calcium supplement from which you can choose and they'll all help boost your body's calcium stores (including calcium citrate/malate, calcium citrate, microcrystalline hydroxyapatite, amino acid chelates, and coral calcium). Calcium carbonate tends to be a popular choice since it's inexpensive. Some calcium carbonate supplements don't dissolve quickly enough to be usable by the body. To check yours, simply put a tablet in a half-cup of vinegar and stir occasionally. It should be completely dissolved after thirty minutes.

If you take iron supplements, don't take your calcium and iron pills at the same time because they compete for absorption. Calcium supplements cause gas or constipation in a small number of people; if you're affected this way, try a few different forms to find one that strengthens your bones without taxing your tummy.

Vitamin D

Following the valid advice to stay out of the sun and apply sunscreen when outside has left the majority of American adults with a vitamin D shortfall. Adding to the vitamin D deficit, scientists now realize that we need even more of this vitamin than previously thought. Why does this matter? Because vitamin D reduces the risk of developing diabetes, rheumatoid arthritis, multiple sclerosis, and cancer, not to mention the "side" benefits of stronger bones and a longer life.[7]

Vitamin D is underappreciated for its crucial role in preventing osteoporosis. This vitamin is needed for the efficient absorption of calcium, which is the principal bone mineral, so if you're going to get enough calcium in your body and keep it there, you have to have enough vitamin D.

The skin uses sunlight to produce vitamin D, so getting a moderate amount of sun exposure every day will provide the body with at least some vitamin D. The skin's ability to manufacture vitamin D decreases with advancing age. In addition, there are concerns that even people who spend time outdoors regularly still might not make enough vitamin D. For example, in a study of people living in Hawaii (who averaged a whopping nearly thirty hours of sun exposure each week), half of the study participants showed a vitamin D deficiency.[8] Increasingly, it is becoming evident that most people, regardless of diet or sun exposure, would benefit from a daily supplement of vitamin D.

During the winter cold and flu season, you definitely don't want to run low on vitamin D. This vitamin is a cheap and effective way to rev up immune defenses and prevent influenza. Scientific evidence shows that achieving adequate vitamin D status reduces your chances of contracting influenza, and if you do get the flu, it will be less severe if your vitamin D levels are higher.

If you are considering a future pregnancy, you'll want to be especially mindful of vitamin D. Many mothers-to-be don't consume enough vitamin D in their diets, which may make it harder for their children to build strong, healthy bones.[9] Supplementing with vitamin D makes sense for pregnant women, considering that, in addition to making healthy bones for both mom and baby, upping vitamin D intake during pregnancy slashes the risk of preeclampsia by about 25 percent.[10]

Getting enough vitamin D may also pay off in a trimmer waistline. The more vitamin D circulating in the bloodstream, the lower a person's body weight. Women with lower levels of vitamin D are sixteen pounds (7 kg) heavier, on average, than women with adequate levels of this sunshine vitamin, according to research.[11]

Supplements of vitamin D come in two forms: vitamin D_2 (ergocalciferol) and vitamin D_3 (cholecalciferol). The first is made from fungus or plant sources and the second comes from animal sources. Go for the D_3 form of this vitamin; it's more effective.

If you already take a multivitamin/mineral supplement, it's likely to provide 200–400 IU of vitamin D. Keep that in mind if you also take a stand-alone vitamin D product. Sun exposure and foods will, of course, also contribute vitamin D to your body's supply, so not all of your vitamin D needs to come from supplements. Good food sources of vitamin D include fish, milk, eggs, and cheese. Your body can make 10,000 IU of vitamin D with twenty to thirty minutes of sun exposure on a sunny day. Sun lovers won't overdose on vitamin D; this vitamin doesn't increase to toxic levels, no matter how much sun exposure you get. The body has some fail-safes in place to guard against excess skin production of this nutrient.

Iron

Iron deficiency is the most common nutritional deficiency in this country. The recommended intake for iron each day is 18 mg for women. Women, in general, are at high risk for iron-deficiency anemia, but your risk goes through the roof during pregnancy and in the postpartum period.

Diagnosing anemia is quick and easy at your doctor's office and treated with iron supplements (you should not supplement with iron if you haven't been diagnosed with iron deficiency). Standard iron tests (either hemoglobin or hematocrit) only show late stages of iron deficiency, called anemia. Not many people are outright anemic, although loads of folks unknowingly have mild or moderate iron deficiency. For this you should ask your doctor to do one of these tests: serum ferritin, serum iron, transferrin saturation, or transferrin receptor test.

The most absorbable form of iron, called *heme* iron, is found in red meat, poultry, and seafood. Nonheme iron is also found in these foods, as well as in dry beans and peas, dark-green leafy vegetables, and molasses. Vitamin C–rich foods or supplements taken with an iron-rich meal boosts iron absorption. On the other hand, coffee and tea may impair iron absorption.

As a supplement, iron is most effective when taken on an empty stomach. However, the most common form of iron supplement, ferrous sulfate, tends to be irritating to the GI tract and may cause cramps, diarrhea, or constipation. Other forms of iron supplements, such as ferrous fumarate, ferrous gluconate, heme-iron concentrate, and iron glycine amino acid chelate are less likely to cause GI side effects.

WHEN SHOULD YOU TAKE SUPPLEMENTS?

The short answer: whenever you can be sure to take your supplements will end up being the best time for you. Dietary supplements that sit forgotten on your countertop won't help you, so choose a convenient time and stick with it. If you're aiming for optimal, though, the longer answer gets a tad more complicated.

Unless the label says otherwise, assume that taking most supplements with food will be a bit better than on an empty stomach. For most people, breakfast or dinnertime ends up being the most opportune time for remembering daily pills. Taking supplements with food improves absorption and minimizes nausea (as sometimes happens when taking a multi on an empty stomach). In particular, taking B-complex vitamins with food will help to avoid queasiness, and calcium absorption improves when it's taken after a meal. Only a few supplements are best taken on an empty stomach, including iron, probiotics, and proteolytic enzymes, such as bromelain or protease. (The small amount of iron in a multivitamin/mineral is fine to take with food, however.)

Keep in mind that alcohol interferes with the absorption of many nutrients, so it's best to take your supplements at a meal that won't include alcohol. Make sure to store your supplements in a cool, dark place, since heat and light may degrade some of the nutrients in a multi.

SUPPLEMENT SAFETY: TOO MUCH OF A GOOD THING?

When it comes to vitamins and minerals, just as *too little* can lead to health problems, so can taking *too much*. Sometimes this happens when people take multiple products with overlapping ingredients—such as a multivitamin, an extra antioxidant, and perhaps a few specialty supplements. Even though each individual product is being used "as directed," the combination may result in a double or triple dose of certain nutrients.

Fortunately, the vast majority of problems stemming from excessive vitamin or mineral intake are simply nuisances, such as skin rash or itching, gastrointestinal upset (diarrhea or constipation), or headache, that resolve themselves when dosages are lowered.

Granted, side effects may occur when taking nutritional supplements, but what's the bigger picture? When it comes down to a risk-benefit analysis, there's no doubt that including supplements in an overall health plan confers more benefits than potential risks. See Appendix: Herb and Dietary Supplement Safety for more information on potential contraindications and risks involved in taking particular supplements.

Beta-carotene

The body converts beta-carotene into vitamin A. At very high doses, it may cause a harmless (and reversible) yellow coloring in the palms of the hands and soles of the feet.
STAY BELOW: 25 mg

Calcium

Calcium is essential for healthy bones, but for those prone to kidney stones, it may raise the risk of stone formation.
STAY BELOW: 1,500 mg

Folic acid

The concern with folic acid is not so much a problem with the nutrient itself but rather that folic acid supplements may mask vitamin B_{12}-related anemia. Folic acid corrects the type of anemia that a vitamin B_{12} deficiency causes. So if a doc tests for vitamin B_{12} deficiency using the common test of checking for anemia, it appears that everything is okay. However, the untreated vitamin B_{12} deficiency could meanwhile be causing nerve damage (which may be permanent).
STAY BELOW: 1,000 mcg

Iron

For this mineral, the potential for harm is greatest for older men and postmenopausal women, and both of these groups generally should *not* supplement with this mineral. Most people will suffer stomach upset from too much iron before any other adverse effects set in, which serves as a clear indicator to lower the supplemental amount.
STAY BELOW: 45 mg (empty stomach) or 60 mg (full stomach)

Magnesium

Too much magnesium may cause loose stools, which explains why the mineral is the active ingredient in many laxatives.
STAY BELOW: 400 mg

Selenium

Taking too much selenium may cause garlic breath, hair loss, skin rashes, and brittle fingernails.
STAY BELOW: 200 mcg

Vitamin A

Too much vitamin A might increase the risk of hip fractures. This potential problem appears to occur at lower dosages than we previously thought. In response, supplement manufacturers have replaced much of the vitamin A in their formulas with beta-carotene. Other signs of too much vitamin A include nausea, vomiting, hair loss, and dry and cracked lips.
STAY BELOW: 1,500 mcg

Vitamin B$_6$

Over time, high doses of this vitamin may cause nerve damage, such as a tingling sensation in the hands and feet.
STAY BELOW: 100 mg

Vitamin C

The safety profile of vitamin C is outstanding; however, people with hemochromatosis (an iron overload disease) shouldn't have extra vitamin C, nor should those susceptible to kidney stones. For anyone, higher doses of vitamin C may cause stomach upset and diarrhea.
STAY BELOW: 2,000 mg

Zinc

While moderate amounts of zinc support a healthy immune system, taking excessive amounts may have the opposite effect, making you more susceptible to infections. However, even moderately high levels may cause nausea. *Note:* It's okay to take extra zinc for a short time, such as using zinc lozenges to treat the common cold.
STAY BELOW: 30 mg

ARE YOU ON THE PILL?

Oral contraceptives are among the most common prescriptions written by doctors; they are also among the most likely drugs to interfere with the body's absorption of numerous nutrients. Major studies show that women taking the Pill would do well to consider taking a variety of dietary supplements.

Do Your Kids Need a Supplement, Too?

A multimultivitamin/mineral is an important safety net for preschoolers and school-age children, but there are other dietary supplements that your child could benefit from, such as these:

Calcium: Kids need calcium primarily to build strong bones. Aim for 800 mg daily for ages four to eight; 1,300 mg daily for ages nine to thirteen.

DHA: This omega-3 fatty acid supports the growing brains of children and calms inflammation. Most kids in the United States don't get enough DHA. Aim for 150 mg of DHA daily.

Probiotics: Beneficial bacteria help with bowel problems (diarrhea and constipation), protect against ear infections, ease eczema, and minimize side effects from antibiotics. Follow label directions, but kids ages six to twelve can generally take one-half of the adult dose, and for under six years old, take one-fourth of the adult dose. Probiotics are particularly important if your child needs to take antibiotics. Give the probiotics during a course of antibiotics and continue afterward for as many days as the antibiotics were used.

Vitamin D: This vitamin is very important for kids' bone health, as well as for the prevention of two biggies of childhood: diabetes and asthma. Most multis provide too little vitamin D, if they have any at all. Look for the vitamin D_3 form (it might be listed as *cholecalciferol* on product labels); D_3 works much better than other forms of vitamin D. Aim for 400 IU per day for your child, which is available in liquid drops.

Lower blood levels of folic acid—one side effect of taking the Pill—are associated with health problems, such as anemia, cervical dysplasia (a precancerous condition of the cervix), headache, fatigue, increased risk of heart disease, and higher risk of breast cancer. If a woman with low levels of folic acid does become pregnant, her unborn child is at much higher risk of numerous birth defects, such as spina bifida. If you are on the Pill, aim for 400 mcg of folic acid daily, the amount generally included in a multivitamin/mineral.

Women on the Pill should take 10–25 mg of vitamin B_6 (which is the amount found in many multis) to guard against the Pill's depletion of this important nutrient. Pill users who feel depressed may consider taking the higher amount of 40 mg per day, to assess whether it relieves their depression.

Too little magnesium—another common Pill side effect—may increase blood pressure, lead to cardiac arrhythmia, promote muscle cramps, and increase the severity of premenstrual syndrome (PMS). Women on the Pill should aim for 300 mg of magnesium daily, which is the amount generally included in a multivitamin/mineral.

CHAPTER 5

Fitting in Exercise

If you've just had a baby, and especially if you're nursing, please don't starve yourself to reach your weight loss goal. Finding time for exercise makes so much more sense—it keeps you strong and healthy, slims and firms your body, and gives you a much-needed mood and morale boost. There's really no downside to breaking a sweat on a regular basis. In fact, with exercise you can get your body back, possibly even in better shape than prekids.

"I started walking with my baby in a stroller to help her take a nap on some days, and then I realized how much getting outside for a walk was helping my outlook and energy on those days," says new mom Ashley. In fact, she kept walking several times a week (adding distance as she got stronger) and by the time her son was nine months old, Ashley was pleasantly surprised to discover that not only could she fit back into her prebaby clothes, but she had lost a few extra pounds as well.

WHEN TO START

The first six weeks with a newborn may be very intense, and not everyone will be ready to jump back into a formal exercise routine right away. In fact, I don't know of any new mom who didn't feel exhausted and overwhelmed at first, and if she claimed not to, I assumed she was lying. These first weeks are the time to pare your to-do list down to the bare minimum. Put all nonessential activities on hold. In other words, baby yourself along with your new baby.

After your baby is born, you can gradually resume exercising, as you feel up to it. In general, a woman with an uncomplicated vaginal delivery should be able to work back to her normal exercise routine by six weeks' postpartum. A good way to ease back into exercise is to start taking brief walks; for most women, it's probably wise to begin a walking regimen in the first week or so after a vaginal delivery. Start small. Even a walk around the block with your baby in a front pack or stroller is a good starting point.

The sooner you start moving your body, the better it will be for you. The first six months after having a baby are the most crucial and predictive of who will lose the baby weight (and keep it off) and who won't.

Working out with other new mothers is a great choice for three reasons: First, a workout buddy makes it more likely that you'll stick to your exercise plan. Second, it's more fun with a partner. Third, you get social time while exercising to combat feelings of loneliness and isolation. Rachel and Shelley certainly found this to be true. "I remember one day I headed out with my screaming, overtired baby to get him to fall asleep and I ran into another new mom (pushing twins in a stroller) whose babies were only weeks apart from my child, and I didn't even know she lived in my neighborhood," says Rachel. "For weeks we had each felt trapped alone at home with crying babies; we soon had a standing date to walk together with our babies. The company was probably even more beneficial than our shared exercise time. It was a real lifesaver," she adds.

Rachel and Shelley found out what women across the country are also discovering: a stroller workout is just about the easiest way to get fit while caring for a baby. Even though you might not have time to eat breakfast or even go to the bathroom without holding your baby, and you probably feel as if you certainly don't have time to go to the gym, you should be able to walk with a stroller. If you don't have a friend to walk with, there are many class options that let you work out with your baby. You can find some through websites, such as strollerfit.com, strollerstrides.com, strollercize.com, and babybootcamp.com.

Starting a New Exercise Routine

1. Choose an activity that you enjoy (walking, hiking, biking, skiing, swimming, whatever), and don't forget that sex itself is a form of exercise (you're welcome, dads)! For beginners, walking is often an ideal choice. You can do it inside (say, at a mall) or outside. You don't have to purchase any special equipment, it doesn't take any special skills or abilities, it has a low risk of injuries, and you can do it alone or with a buddy.

2. Don't push too hard at first. Start slowly so that your body gets used to exercise and you aren't too sore to continue.

3. Keep convenience in mind. If you want to join a gym, choose one close to your home or office and check to see if it has child care. Make sure you have exercise options that don't depend on a certain type of weather. You don't want any easy excuses to skip your exercise that day.

4. Spice up your routine. Don't sabotage yourself by only doing one class at the gym or using only one exercise machine at home. Rotate through different activities so that boredom doesn't stop you from exercising.

5. Work out with a buddy. This will help keep you motivated and lessen the chance that you'll skip the workout.

STRETCHING

The daily responsibilities of your new job as mom may be pretty rough on your body. There's the constant lifting (car seat, stroller, baby, etc.), hunching over to breast-feed, and pacing the halls for hours at night with a crying baby. All the while, your breasts weigh a few extra pounds and your abdominal muscles are weakened. The end result? You likely feel tired and achy all the time. Gentle stretching can make a big difference in countering these stresses of new motherhood.

Stretching is all too easily overlooked. It doesn't take long, and, for the time invested, can give you a great buffer against injury, as well. You can stretch between sets at the gym, at the end of a cardio activity, or

Check Your Intensity

The American Heart Association (as well as many health experts) recommends thirty minutes of moderate-intensity exercise five days a week. But how do you know if you're at "moderate" intensity? San Diego State University researchers determined that women who walk at a brisk pace of approximately 100 steps a minute reach moderate intensity.[1] That ends up being 3,000 steps in a thirty-minute exercise session. Use a pedometer to check that you're at this pace. Alternatively, if you exercise hard enough to feel your heart and breathing rate increase, but you're still able to chat using full sentences, then you've likely entered the moderate zone. Want another way to know if your walking speed is fast enough? If you match your stride to "Stayin' Alive" by the Bee Gees, you'll be walking 100 steps per minute.

while sitting on the family room floor playing with your baby. Remember to hold each stretch (without bouncing or straining) for at least ten seconds. If you have the best of intentions, but never seem to make the time to stretch, maybe you'd find a yoga or pilates DVD more to your liking.

SUMMER EXERCISE ADVICE

Working up a sweat exercising during the summer months literally drains your body of water. Avoiding dehydration is especially important if you are breast-feeding. While filling back up can be as easy as turning on the kitchen faucet, sometimes other beverages work even better than plain water, especially when your exercise bouts get longer or more intense.

Sports drinks rank above water for rehydrating the body in two key ways: quicker absorption and the flavoring and electrolyte content encourage you to drink more. One study found that even low-fat chocolate milk works as well as common sports drinks to refuel exercise-weary muscles, probably because of a great ratio of fluid, carbs, and protein. No matter what beverage you choose before, during, or after working out, drinking it chilled will send it through the stomach faster and get it absorbed more quickly.

It's just a fact: most athletes don't drink enough during exercise to keep up with sweat losses, but you can train yourself to become a better drinker. Make it easy by keeping water or other drinks on hand, and remember to take a swig whenever you notice thirst.

Pollution is generally the worst in the summer. If you enjoy outside exercise, minimize your exposure to pollutants by not exercising during rush hours and switching to an indoor exercise on hot, humid, windless days when pollution is at its highest.

WINTER EXERCISE ADVICE

As winter settles in, it's tempting to settle into your couch, nestling with your new baby for a three-month rest. Granted, it may be more difficult to stay active during the winter months, but there are ways to make it more tolerable, whether you brave the outdoors or break a sweat inside.

Burning Calories

Ever wondered just how long it takes to burn off a sweet treat you devoured in a momentary breakdown of willpower? This chart is based on a 150-pound (68-kg) person; someone weighing less will burn fewer calories and someone weighing more will burn more calories for each hour of physical activity.

ACTIVITY	CALORIES BURNED PER HOUR	ACTIVITY	CALORIES BURNED PER HOUR
Aerobics, low impact	396	Running (12 min/mile)	576
Aerobics, high impact	504	Stair-stepping machine	432
Aerobics, water	288	Stretching	288
Bicycle, stationary	504	Walking (15 min/mile)	324
Circuit training	576	Weight-lifting	216
Elliptical	648		

Once you've gotten yourself motivated on a cold winter day to stick to your exercise goals, the next step is to dress for success. Layering is key for winter workouts, because it is the most effective way to stay warm and has the added advantage of allowing you to remove layers as you warm up. Remember: the layer next to your skin should be one that keeps away moisture and your outermost layer should have some reflective material so that you can be seen on gloomier winter days. Give your feet special attention, especially on wet, cold days. The warmer your feet are, the warmer your body will be.

Warming up properly is essential during winter months, but you need to be careful not to perform any stretches if your body temperature has dropped. Before you do any stretching, you should bring up your body temperature so that the muscles are warm and not as prone to injury. You could walk ten to fifteen minutes on cold days to warm the body up, and don't forget that a period of cooldown and stretching at the end is very important, as well. It's a good idea to add on clothing layers or go indoors during cooldown and stretching, so you don't become chilled and more susceptible to injuries.

Seven Tips for Winter Weather Exercise

- Join a health club to keep active despite the crummy weather (look for one with child care).
- Keep walking, either outdoors bundled up or indoors at a shopping mall or on an indoor track or treadmill.
- Swim laps.
- Buy (and use!) home exercise equipment.
- Buy some exercise DVDs, or check out some from the library so you don't get bored with the same ones.
- Perform miniworkouts during commercial breaks of the TV shows you watch: jumping jacks, skipping rope, or weight-lifting. If you have a treadmill, you could walk throughout one program.
- Enjoy the winter season: try cross-country skiing or snowshoeing.

Surprisingly, winter exercisers need to think about overheating as a result of overdressing. In fact, the temperature may be tropical inside a running suit. Dehydration is an oft-forgotten hazard of the winter months, since exercisers don't feel as thirsty in winter as they do in summer. Keep yourself hydrated by drinking before, during, and after workouts. Not drinking enough even raises the risk of hypothermia.

Outdoor workouts in cold weather are not for everyone, however. It would be best to move workouts indoors for exercisers who have asthma or other conditions that compromise the upper respiratory system because cold winter air (especially when it's dry) is a common asthma trigger and may cause symptoms in the majority of asthmatics. If that's not feasible, those with asthma should drink plenty of fluids before and after exercise to keep the airways moist, wear a scarf over the mouth and nose so that the air is warmed before being breathed in, and ensure a proper warm-up and cooldown.

When the weather is just too nasty for you (and your child) to venture out, there are a lot of options for getting your heart rate up inside your own home. For example, you can jog in place or jump-rope or even shadowbox for five minutes, do some squats with no weights, move on to lunges and push-ups, then jump-rope again for another five minutes. Try alternating weight work and cardio—five minutes each. This keeps the boredom level down and the heart rate up.

Winter may be the perfect time to join a gym or health club. Among the best low-impact exercises for beginners at the gym are the recumbent bike (good for people with bad backs), the treadmill, and the elliptical machine. All these cardio machines have resistance variability so you can up the intensity as your fitness improves. Weight training is an important part of overall fitness, but beginners should have a professional at the gym walk them through a workout, demonstrating proper form for each of the exercises.

HYDRATION

A good workout works up a sweat—and that means your body is losing water. Even with a mild level of dehydration, you probably aren't playing your best game. Aside from the obvious feeling of thirst, dehydration hampers the ability to concentrate, makes you feel fatigued at a lower intensity of work than you otherwise would, increases physiological strain, and impairs both aerobic and anaerobic sports performance.

Many athletes, particularly those who live in warm climates, are unwittingly living in a state of chronic mild dehydration.[2] The problem can often be traced back to the quirky physiological fact that your body doesn't send out the signal of thirst until you've already lost quite a bit of water. By the time you want to wet your whistle, about 2 percent of your body weight in water is already spent. This 2 percent threshold of lost water is about where exercise performance starts to noticeably decline.[3]

Staying well-hydrated should actually start before you start exercising; drinking one to two glasses of water in the two hours before exercising will help prepare your body for the work ahead. Once you are actively engaged in physical activity, don't forget to take water breaks to drink about half a cup (100 ml) every fifteen to twenty minutes. Finally, remember to drink several glasses of water in the hours after exercise to replenish water that was lost as a result of sweating.

One easy way to gauge your hydration status is to take note of the color of your urine. It will be a pale yellow if you are well hydrated. The darker your urine, the more dehydrated your body is, and the more water you need to drink to correct your water deficit.

Water is a cheap and effective rehydration choice. Even though plain H_2O does the trick in most scenarios, there are advantages to sports drinks. Research shows that people drink greater quantities when the beverage is flavored. The added carbohydrates in sports drinks also boost consumption and improve the absorption of the fluids. But the best trick of all to encourage fluid intake is to simply make sure that whatever you have with you is kept cold. Cool drinks are much more likely to be consumed than warm ones or those at room temperature.

WOMEN AND ANEMIA

Of all the essential vitamins and minerals, iron holds a place of special importance for the athlete because it transports oxygen to and within

Determine Your Sweat Loss

One of the main goals of drinking water or other fluids before, during, and after exercise is to replace water lost through sweating. But sweat rates vary among athletes, so how much water do you need to compensate for your amount of sweating?

STEP 1: Weigh yourself nude before exercising.

STEP 2: Exercise as you normally do, while keeping track of how much water or other fluids you consume during the workout.

STEP 3: Again, weigh yourself nude.

The difference in weight before and after exercising is how much water you lost as a result of exercising. Of course, you'll need to adjust for the amount you drank during the workout.

For example, if you weighed one pound (0.5 kg) less after exercising than you did before, and you drank 16 ounces (454 g) during exercise (which weighs about a pound [0.5 kg]), then you lost about two pounds (1 kg) of sweat. Two pounds (1 kg) of water is about four 8-ounce (227 g) glasses, so you'll want to drink that much (or as much as you can tolerate) every time you exercise. You may divide it up, such as 8 ounces (227 g) every fifteen minutes.

the muscle cells. Iron-deficient people get pooped during a workout because their bodies are starved for oxygen.

Iron deficiency is the most common nutritional deficiency in this country and athletes (especially female athletes) are particularly at risk because they have higher daily iron losses. In the general population, an estimated 11–13 percent have the preanemic condition of iron deficiency, while 3–5 percent of young women have outright iron-deficiency anemia.[4]

Meanwhile, in one study, 20 percent of athletic women showed signs of iron depletion, 10 percent had iron deficiency, and 10 percent had iron-deficiency anemia.[5] Other research results are even more dire, finding that 26 percent of female endurance athletes were deficient in iron.[6] Exercising women who are iron-deficient will notice slower exercise times, reduced endurance, muscle soreness, fatigue, lethargy, irritability, and poor concentration.

Overall, studies of both men and women, involving a variety of sporting disciplines, all concur that athletes are more likely than the general population to develop iron deficiency. In fact, the problems that athletes have with this mineral are so well known in the medical community that it has been dubbed "sports anemia." Undue fatigue is often the first noticeable sign of iron deficiency; if you've found yourself dragging through what used to be a routine workout, you should have your iron status evaluated by a health care practitioner.

Although few people are anemic, a large number of people are somewhat deficient in the mineral iron. The iron tests commonly used by doctors (either hemoglobin or hematocrit) are best-suited to show the severe iron deficiency of anemia and don't reveal mild or moderate deficiencies. If you ask your doctor for a different test, such as a serum ferritin, serum iron, transferrin saturation, or transferrin receptor test, you can find out if you have a less severe deficiency of iron.

Aerobic activities, and especially those relying on endurance, are the most likely to be impacted by sports anemia. The more active and devoted an athlete, the lower that athlete's iron level tends to be. Within the category of endurance activities, runners seem to be the most likely to be affected. The "traumatic" actions involved in running are thought to trigger the destruction of red blood cells (one of the prime homes of iron in the body).

If your body has adequate iron stores to draw from, extra iron won't make you perform better. However, for those with less than optimal stores, iron supplementation has a clear and well-established benefit. For example, when iron-deficient elite athletes were supplemented with iron (100 mg of elemental iron twice daily) for three months, there was a clear increase in aerobic performance capacity, compared to a placebo group.[7] Similarly, when nonathletes with iron deficiency took iron supplements or a placebo, those taking the iron for six weeks showed much greater improvements in cycle times.[8]

The recommended intake for iron each day is 18 mg for women. The need for iron is estimated to be 30 percent greater in anyone engaging in regular, intense exercise. These amounts may be tough to get for many people, since even the best food source of iron—red meat—only supplies about 3 mg per 3-ounce (85-g) serving. People with iron deficiency are given much higher amounts of iron as a supplement to replenish their body stores, generally 100 mg per day until the deficiency is corrected. (Work with a doctor before consuming a high dose of iron, however.) Iron supplements can make a big difference, but it is a good idea to have a quick blood test to assess your iron status before starting supplementation. Excessive iron may damage the liver and has, in some studies, been linked to a higher risk of certain cancers and heart attack.

EXERCISE INJURIES

There is no question that exercise is an important component of good health. But there are times that injuries occur as a direct result of exercise. This happens more often than you might think: seven million Americans receive medical attention for sports- and recreation-related injuries every year.[9] Fortunately, many injuries are fairly minor; for example, strains and sprains account for 31 percent of sports injuries.

There are steps you can take to minimize your chances of getting hurt. First and foremost, warm up before you exercise. This can be as simple as a few minutes of slow walking or using light weights. Warming up increases blood flow to the muscles and boosts your metabolic rate in preparation for the work ahead. Likewise, it is helpful to cool down after you exercise. Simply ease down the intensity of your activity for the last five minutes. This gives your body a chance to adjust and promotes the removal of lactic acid (a cause of muscle soreness).

Don't forget the basics, such as choosing well-fitting shoes that are designed for your activity, learning the proper techniques for your chosen sport, and wearing the appropriate safety equipment for the sport, like a helmet for biking and goggles for racquetball. Most importantly, listen to your body and don't overexert yourself or work out beyond your capability.

Too Late—Now What?

The RICE procedure is the gold standard for treating sports injuries. However, if pain or swelling worsens after twenty-four hours, consult a physician.

Rest the injured area.

Ice the injured area for twenty-minute intervals, with forty minutes of non-ice time in between each session.

Compress the injured area with an ACE bandage or similar wrap.

Elevate the injured area above heart level.

WOMEN'S UNIQUE SPORTS INJURY RISK

If you're an active woman, your knee may be a ticking time bomb. Women are up to eight times more likely than men to injure a ligament in their knees during sports activities—a type of injury that is woefully hard to treat and often sets the stage for osteoarthritis later in life. This injury-prone ligament, called the anterior cruciate ligament (ACL), is positioned deep within the knee, where it serves as the fulcrum of stability for the knee, connecting the shin bone to the thigh bone.

A wider pelvic girdle (which recently came in handy when you gave birth) appears to be one culprit in making women's ACL so vulnerable; the wider pelvic girdle causes the location of the knee to be at a slightly wider angle. This wider angle is a source of stress on the ACL. Hormones also play a role. Studies have found estrogen and progesterone receptors on the ACL. These hormones have been shown to make the muscles, ligaments, and joints more lax—and more prone to injuries— during both ovulatory and menstrual cycles. Women who take oral contraceptives have fewer hormone fluctuations and a correspondingly lower risk of ACL injury.

Most commonly, ACL injuries are seen in players of sports like soccer, volleyball, basketball, skiing, or football that involve deceleration, twisting, or jumping. You might hear a "pop" at the time of injury, the pain could be severe, and the knee will generally swell up in the first few hours. The standard injury treatment of RICE—rest, ice, compression, and elevation—is called for in these cases. If the knee continues to give out and feel unstable after recovery would be expected, surgical reconstruction might be necessary.

Unfortunately, the long-term prognosis for an ACL injury is dismal. One study found that twelve years after women injured their ACL, more than half had developed osteoarthritis in that knee and three-quarters of the women reported that the knee continued to be painful.[10] Since the women were only an average of thirty-one years old when their knees were injured, ACL injuries tend to result in young women with the knees of old women.

There are a few dietary supplements that help promote the healing of any soft-tissue injury, including ACL knee injuries. At the top of the list are the enzymes bromelain and papain (from papaya). These enzymes reduce inflammation and aid the repair of injured tissue. In addition, vitamin C and zinc both play crucial roles in repairing connective-tissue wounds, so it would be prudent to supplement with these while healing from an ACL injury. Glucosamine sulfate and chondroitin sulfate are supplements that supply the body with some important building blocks for repairing ligaments; they are also worth a try. Finally, topical use of horse chestnut gel might also aid in the healing process.

Since the ACL has very poor healing potential, prevention should be on every active woman's mind. There are several training methods that you can incorporate to reduce your risk of an ACL injury. You'd be smart to listen closely, because training regimens with ACL health in mind could cut the number of injuries by as much as 80 percent.

- Strengthen your hamstrings. A top priority is to build strength in your hamstring muscle because this takes some stress off the ACL.

- Practice safer jumping and landing techniques. Women tend to bend their knees less than men when landing from a jump; this ups the stress on the knee joint. Practicing jumps that end with a bent-knee landing has been documented to help prevent injuries.

- Use a different position for quick turning maneuvers. Women are more likely to pivot and turn in a more upright position than men. Practicing maneuvers in a crouching position (with a slight bend at the knee and hip) has a protective effect on knee health.

NUTRITION FOR ATHLETIC MOMS

Expecting the most from your body means demanding the best from your diet. Selecting a variety of low-fat, minimally processed foods— such as whole-grain breads and cereals, fruits, vegetables, cooked dried beans and peas, low-fat milk products—together with small amounts of extra-lean meat, chicken, and fish, is essential to lifelong health and fitness.

Besides training, nutrition is the most important influence on exercise performance. An adequate number of calories, carbohydrates, protein, and even dietary fat and water are necessary for a healthy body, and especially for an athlete's body.

Literally, every bite counts for the athlete, because vitamin and mineral needs often increase faster than calorie needs. Unfortunately, many athletes do not always eat the optimal diet. Nutritional surveys reveal that many exercisers—from weekend warriors to professional athletes—consume diets low in vitamin C, vitamin B_1, vitamin B_6, calcium,

---

Gender Differences

The bodies of male and female athletes react differently during long-duration exercise. Men's muscles rely on carbohydrates to keep moving, while women's muscles derive more expended energy from fats.

What this means is that carbohydrate bars and drinks might be more effective for men than women, as a way to increase endurance. In addition, this gender difference in fuel usage might explain why "carbo-loading" has been documented to work for men, but not women. One piece of good news for female athletes, though, is that, after a long, hard workout, women recover faster from exercise-induced muscle damage than men do.

chromium, iron, magnesium, and zinc. Even marginal deficiencies of these essential nutrients can jeopardize general health, reduce resistance to colds and infections, and interfere with exercise, resulting in reduced endurance, fatigue, or an inability to improve performance.

For a great start to a healthy body and competitive performance, eat a balanced diet that provides optimal amounts of all the essential nutrients and supplement to fill in the gaps where the diet falls short.

Carbohydrates

Carbohydrates are an important fuel for all types of exercise. Carbs are the primary energy source for stop-and-start sports, such as tennis and volleyball, and the kindling fuel necessary to ignite fat burning in aerobic sports, such as running, cycling, and swimming.

What is eaten immediately before exercise is also important. An easily digested carbohydrate snack (such as fruit and a bagel), eaten one to three hours before exercising, can boost blood sugar levels, and this helps spare glycogen. By contrast, sugary foods, such as candy bars or soda pop, should be avoided just before exercise, since concentrated sugars can lower blood sugar and impair athletic endurance.

Even what you eat after exercising is important. A high-carbohydrate snack, eaten fifteen to thirty minutes after a workout, helps restore glycogen for the next exercise session.

Protein

Water bathes the muscles and carbohydrates fuels them, but protein serves as the bricks and mortar for building muscle. Protein allows muscles to contract, grow in size, and increase in strength.

The most plentiful food sources of protein are meat, poultry, fish, dairy products, legumes, and grains. After eating, proteins in these foods are broken down into their component parts—which are called amino acids—and then absorbed and used by the body. The body itself can make many amino acids, except for nine or ten "essential" amino acids that must be obtained from the diet. Eating a variety of protein-rich foods ensures that your body has access to the many amino acids that contribute to a strong, capable, athletic physique. Frequent exercisers have an increased need for dietary protein, compared to the protein needs of the average person. However, it is rare that an athlete will actually be lacking in protein, since the average American already consumes two to three times the daily requirement for protein.

Protein in excess of body needs is either stored as fat or broken down. A little extra protein is harmless. However, excessive protein intake may damage the kidneys and liver and result in dehydration and even mineral deficiencies. The key is to consume enough, without consuming too much.

WHERE TO FIND PROTEIN

FOOD	PROTEIN (GRAMS)
Skim milk, 1 cup (200 ml)	8
Yogurt, 1 cup (200 ml)	8
Chicken breast, 1 ounce (28 g)	7
Turkey, 1 ounce (28 g)	7
Tuna, 1 ounce (28 g)	7
Rice, 2/3 cup (133 ml) (cooked)	6
Potato, 1 small	3
Bread, 1 slice	3
Pasta, 1/2 cup (100 ml) (cooked)	3
Banana, 1 medium	2
Apple, 1 small	1

MULTIVITAMINS = MULTI BENEFITS

Multivitamin/mineral supplements are taken by about 50 percent of athletes.[11] A multi is not necessarily a true ergogenic aid. That is, it doesn't appear to work in a direct fashion to make an athlete stronger, faster, or better. However, just as you can't build the best home on a rotten foundation, a multi can ensure that your body's foundation is solid—so your body is receptive to the benefits of athletic training.

The typical once-a-day multi supplement provides up to 100 percent of the recommended amount of many of the essential vitamins and minerals. This type of supplement is very safe to use and serves as a form of nutritional insurance. A separate supplement of minerals (such as calcium, magnesium, and zinc) might be necessary, since these are bulkier nutrients that take up so much space that a multi would be too big to swallow if it contained enough of these.

Some nutrition experts contend that a daily multi is simply unnecessary if good food choices are made, and even go as far as to discourage the use of a multi, fearing that it may be used as a substitute for healthful food choices. However, far from using the multi to "make up" for a poor diet, athletes who take a multi supplement have a healthier diet. Individuals who supplement their diet eat more vitamin- and mineral-rich foods. It's clear that multi supplement users are "supplementing" their good food choices, not trying to replace them.

All adults—athletes or couch potatoes alike—can benefit from a multi. But athletes should keep in mind a few nutrients that are particularly important to have in a multi. For starters, the B-complex vitamins are needed for energy production and the athlete will require more B-complex vitamins than the average Joe. Vitamins C and E are also crucial for athletes, since these vitamins counteract the free radicals that are generated during exercise. Key minerals, such as magnesium and zinc, are also needed during hard training.

EXERCISE AND FREE RADICALS

Strenuous exercise increases the production of free radicals, which can damage muscle tissue and result in inflammation and aching muscles. Exercising in cities or smoggy areas also increases exposure to free radicals.

Fortunately, the body's natural defense system of antioxidants, including vitamin C, the carotenoids, and vitamin E, neutralize free radicals before they can damage the body. Regular exercise increases the efficiency of the antioxidant defense system, but an extra boost of antioxidant vitamins may be needed in older or untrained individuals, or athletes who are undertaking an especially vigorous training protocol or athletic event.

SPORTS BARS

Sports nutrition bars meet a lot of different needs for exercising moms. A sports bar may be a quick pick-me-up before a workout, a way to restore energy supplies after exercise, or even a meal substitute on a busy day.

Sports bars certainly have come a long way from their origin as a niche product developed by a running enthusiast and his nutritionist wife. There are numerous nutrition bars on the market today, but they generally fall into one of three categories:

1. High-carbohydrate bars that are designed as a concentrated energy source

2. High-protein bars that are geared to building muscle mass and controlling weight

3. Meal replacement bars that aim to provide a balanced array of nutrients

The high-carbohydrate nutrition bars—generally dubbed "energy" bars—typically provide 100–300 calories in the form of carbohydrates (although there will be some protein, fat, vitamins, and minerals tossed in, as well). These powerhouses of carbohydrates are an efficient way for endurance athletes to meet their energy needs before exercise. Sports bars may also be great after exercise to replenish glycogen stores. Glycogen, the form of glucose (simple carbohydrates) stored in the muscles and liver, is converted to blood glucose to provide energy for physical exertion.

Protein bars commonly contain protein derived from whey. One reason for this is that whey protein is naturally rich in branched-chain amino acids, which are used by the body for muscle building and muscle repair. Soy protein is another popular protein source that is well regarded for building and maintaining muscle mass. Some protein bars contain gelatin hydrolysate, which is a source of the amino acids glycine and proline. These two amino acids have been studied for their role in building strong connective tissue.

Meal-replacement bars may be a healthy snack for exercising moms to help cover all the nutrient needs of the day. These bars generally provide the most calories of all the nutrition bars. Often, these are a 40:30:30 bar, meaning that 40 percent of the calories are carbohydrates, 30 percent are protein, and 30 percent are fat.

Whichever bar you select, make sure that you are eating it at the right time. Sports bars should be eaten one hour before exercise; they may also be eaten after exercise, of course, but do not consume the bars during exercise because they could trigger stomach upset, and since they require water for digestion they could pull water out of muscle tissue. In addition, they are absorbed more slowly than a sports drink or sports gel—which would be the better choice for during-exercise use. The only time that an athlete might benefit from a sports bar during exercise would be for an extended event (lasting longer than two hours). Even so, only the high-carbohydrate sports bars would be appropriate at such a time.

Another important tip is to make sure to drink 8–12 ounces (227–340 g) of water for each sports nutrition bar you consume. Drinking water is even more important when you choose a high-protein bar that contains glycerol. Not only is water an ergogenic aid (meaning it enhances your performance) in its own right, but drinking water is important to reduce the risk of stomach discomfort that is sometimes associated with protein bars and also to maximize the hydration effects of glycerol.

Just about any snack that provides a couple of hundred calories is going to give results, compared to trying to be active on an empty stomach. Any fuel is better than no fuel. In fact, even a candy bar eaten five minutes before exercise improves performance when compared to having eaten nothing. And sports bars "raise the bar" even higher than candy bars or other similar snacks by providing the right balance of nutrients for the job.

POSTWORKOUT RECOVERY

What you eat or take as a supplement after exercise also counts. Post-workout supplements may shorten recovery time and help athletes reach their personal best.

Muscle damage and inflammation that develops after a strenuous workout is not just a sign of hard work, but also the result of out-of-control free radicals damaging the muscles.[12] Fortunately, regular athletic training primes the antioxidant defenses to face the challenge of extra free radicals. However, those who don't work out regularly probably don't have the heightened internal defenses needed to face down the extra free radicals. In which case, supplementing with antioxidants may counteract the exercise-induced free radical onslaught. The research is particularly plentiful for vitamin C and vitamin E, both of which speed muscle recovery after workouts.

Pyruvate, which is a compound formed in the body as carbohydrates and protein are converted into energy, functions in the body as another antioxidant to inhibit the production of free radicals.[13] In addition, supplements of pyruvate may improve exercise endurance. For example, several clinical trials show that supplementing with pyruvate improves exercise endurance in individuals starting an exercise program.[14]

After an intense bout of exercise (such as a marathon), the immune system's ability to fight off germs is compromised, which results in higher than expected rates of upper respiratory infections in high-level athletes. Quercetin, an antioxidant bioflavonoid found in apples, onions, and tea, has been shown to counteract this effect. Intense exercisers who supplement with quercetin have lower rates of infection than those who don't take this antioxidant.[15] Do not take quercetin during pregnancy.

The amino acid L-carnitine primarily resides in high-energy body tissues (such as muscles), where it plays a crucial role in the production of energy. How much high-intensity exercise the muscles can perform depends, in part, on the availability of L-carnitine. Studies in athletes indicate that supplementation with this nutrient might improve athletic performance, such as by lessening postexercise lactate levels and improving recovery from exercise stress.[16]

Drinking tart cherry juice lessens postexercise pains and muscle soreness, as well as curtailing recovery time after a strenuous bout of exercise.[17] Anthocyanins, the same compound that contribute to the rich red color of cherries, serve as an anti-inflammatory agent in cherries and cherry extract.

Enzyme supplements can be quite useful for anyone who has overdone it with exercise and subsequently develops sore, inflamed muscles and other soft tissues. The enzymes bromelain and papain (from papaya) promote the healing of soft tissues, such as injuries from exercising too hard. These enzymes reduce inflammation and aid the repair of injured tissue. Do not use papain during pregnancy because of a slight risk of uterine contractions.

The herb arnica contains sesquiterpene lactones, which subdue inflammation and ease pain. Arnica in cream or gel form can be used on bruises, strains, or other soft-tissue and joint ailments to provide pain relief and minimize swelling. When arnica gel was compared to an ibuprofen gel in a group of 204 adults with joint pain, the arnica was found to work as well as the conventional pain reliever for easing pain and improving joint function, yet there were fewer side effects with the arnica.[18]

CHAPTER 6

Rediscovering Beauty Basics

Has your "pregnancy glow" been replaced by acne, stretch marks, and spider veins? Hey, that's not a fair trade at all. Having a baby sure does a number on your looks, not to mention how that little one eats up any free time that could be spent on personal care. "I think it was a full two years into mommyhood (with two babies very close together) before I got back to a morning beauty routine, which had been replaced with a frantic swipe of lipstick as I held a fussing baby on my hip," says Carrie. "When I finally scheduled that time into my day—to dry and style my hair and put on makeup—I couldn't believe how much better it made my outlook on life."

Finding the time and energy in your daily schedule to pay a little attention to beauty pays off in many ways. For Jennifer, a mom of twins, putting herself back on the list of priorities took a nudge from an awkward job interview: "At a follow-up interview after I had my twins, I happened to read the interviewer's observation (that I wasn't supposed to see), noting that I looked unprofessional. Wow, did that hit home! In a flash, I realized how I had let fashion and looks fall away after having children. It was a wake-up call, and after that I bought better clothes, got my eyebrows waxed, highlighted my hair, and started wearing makeup again. It's been fun to reawaken that part of myself."

SKIN

Your skin is the first thing that others notice about you; not surprisingly, we all would like our skin to be clear and radiant. If you're an average-size adult, you have twenty-one square feet (1.95 m²) of skin, weighing about nine pounds (4 kg) and containing more than eleven miles (18 km) of blood vessels. Vibrant skin is an outer indication of inner health, since how the skin looks mirrors the health of the rest of the body. Nourishing the body from the inside with wholesome nutrition lays the groundwork for a radiant complexion. A deficiency of any nutrient can have a detrimental effect on skin's appearance. As such, a daily multivitamin/mineral supplement helps you cover your nutritional bases.

Having a baby tends to accelerate and magnify any skin changes. Suddenly, you're seeing lines, marks, and imperfections that didn't seem to be there before. Perhaps prebaby you got by just fine washing your face with a bar of soap. That might not be good enough anymore. If

Skin Must-Do's

Put your best face forward by making these healthy skin choices:

- Don't smoke. If not for your overall health and your child's sake, at least quit to avoid the extra wrinkles smoking guarantees to send your way.

- Wear sunscreen whenever you go out in the sun (and, yes, daily errands count—it's not just for a day at the beach). Sunscreen of at least SPF 15 (SPF 30's better) ranks as the number one anti-aging product, hands down.

- Avoid sun exposure between 10 a.m. and 4 p.m. and don't even consider going to a tanning salon. Ultraviolet light (from the sun or a tanning bed) is the number one contributor to prematurely old-looking skin.

- Drink plenty of water to keep your skin hydrated.

you're noticing some skin changes, it might be a good time to switch over to a mild cleanser. This doesn't have to mean a fancy, expensive cleanser. There are plenty of quality cleansers at any drugstore. If your cleanser makes your skin feel tight after you wash it, that's a sign that it's not gentle enough—get a different one.

Now that your face is clean, it's probably also time to use a moisturizer if you aren't using one already. When skin is dry, even fine lines start to look an awful lot like wrinkles! Apply moisturizer at night; that's when the skin repairs itself. Choose a moisturizer that feels light and is quickly absorbed into your skin.

If you really want to fight against the hands of time (which somehow seem to accelerate postbaby), think about adding in an anti-aging serum to your skin care routine. One with antioxidants (such as vitamin C, alpha-lipoic acid, vitamin E, or selenium) may help boost skin's defenses against damaging free radicals.

Value of Antioxidants

Wrinkled, sagging skin is a hallmark of advancing years (and sleepless nights don't help). But you can fight the march of time, as written across your face, by understanding the enemy. Free radicals, such as oxygen fragments, are marauding molecules that wreak havoc on the cells of the body in a misguided pursuit of stability.

Free radicals are unstable because they have an unpaired or "extra" electrical charge that causes them to seek out other substances in the body to bond with in order to neutralize themselves. Unfortunately, this can cause yet another free radical to be created, thus initiating a chain reaction.

Free radicals are formed in our bodies as a byproduct of the necessary actions of breathing oxygen and burning food for energy. Free radicals are also lurking in air pollution, tobacco smoke, ultraviolet (UV) sun rays, and rancid fats. The targets of free radical attacks are often the fatty membranes that surround cells, but other body components are also damaged by free radicals.

The body is faced with hundreds of thousands of free radical "hits" each day; it's a wonder we can survive this onslaught at all. But the reason our bodies have some success in forestalling free radical damage is an intricate defense system composed of antioxidant vitamins, minerals, and enzymes.

Free radicals may damage the skin's appearance and contribute to an older-looking face in several ways. When the skin's structural proteins—such as collagen or elastin—are attacked, skin loses its elasticity and firm, youthful appearance. Antioxidants, such as vitamin C, vitamin E, the carotenoids, selenium, and many bioflavonoids, protect the skin from this damage.

The more time you spend in the sun, the more important this antioxidant skin protection becomes, since the skin's supply of antioxidants is depleted during sun exposure. For example, beta-carotene decreases the skin's susceptibility to sunburn, particularly reddening and inflammation, and another carotenoid, lycopene, sacrifices itself so that UV rays don't injure the skin.[1] Carotenoids work even better when combined with other antioxidants, such as vitamin E or vitamin C. As the diversity of antioxidants increases, so does their free radical–fighting ability.

Regularly drinking green tea or supplementing with EGCG (the main antioxidant in green tea) also protects against sun damage, as well as reducing the risk of skin cancer.[2] Green tea extract even provides skin protection when applied topically to the surface of the skin.

For skin that has already been damaged by excessive sun exposure, the mineral silicon might offer a reprieve by improving elasticity and suppleness. According to double-blind research involving fifty women with sun-damaged skin, supplementing with either 10 mg of silicon (in the proprietary form of choline-stabilized orthosilicic acid) or a placebo daily for five months resulted in significant improvements to skin roughness and elasticity in those taking the silicon.[3]

Battling Acne

"After continuously being either pregnant or nursing for four years solid, when I weaned my last child, the hormone changes triggered the worst acne breakout of my life," shares Sara. "Even as a teenager I had fairly clear skin; this was the worst my skin had ever looked in my entire life and it went on for a few months. I tried some new facial cleansers, which helped a bit. But mostly I just needed to wait out the hormone flux."

The culprit in acne breakouts like the one Sara experienced is the hormone roller coaster you've been on since pregnancy. Surging hormones ramp up oil-gland production. If you were plagued with pimples in your teenage years and/or with PMS, then you're more likely to get postbaby zits as well. Console yourself with this: acne will not last forever. When your hormones settle down (usually within a few months after giving birth or weaning), your face will go back to normal. In the meantime, care for your skin by washing with a mild cleanser twice a day and using the usual arsenal of anti-acne products.

Aside from the well-known advice to cleanse the face, there is some evidence that supplementing with zinc will help lessen breakouts. For women with PMS-related flare-ups, taking vitamin B_6 (50 mg daily) may be beneficial. In addition, applying tea tree oil (5 percent) to afflicted areas may help resolve breakouts. Beta-carotene supplements may also help you zap the zits, while others report success with supplements of vitamin C, bioflavonoids, vitamin E, calcium, zinc, or brewer's yeast.

Stretch Marks

During pregnancy, your uterus grows an incredible amount and the skin of the abdomen often pays the price with red streaks called stretch marks. They may also develop on your buttocks, breasts, and thighs. About half of women will have them during and after pregnancy. Take heart: they will fade significantly in the six months to a year after you give birth, leaving you with faint silvery-white streaks. Unfortunately, none of the creams and lotions touted to fix stretch marks will do very much. You just have to wait for them to fade.

Varicose Veins

Aside from being a cosmetic issue, varicose veins are a health concern, since they indicate impaired valve function. Improperly working valves allow blood to accumulate in the veins, stretch them out of shape, and leave you with swollen, bulging blue veins in your legs. Pregnancy ups your risk for this less-than-appealing condition because the extra blood in your body during pregnancy tends to pool in the legs, enlarging the veins. To make matters worse, the weight of your growing uterus puts extra pressure on the veins in your legs. Pregnancy hormones tend to promote relaxation in the walls of veins. All this adds up to a case of varicose veins for many pregnant women. Varicose veins may cause an achy, heavy feeling as well as leg cramps, itchiness, and throbbing. Sitting or standing in one place exacerbates the symptoms.

Compression stockings (also known as support hose) help the aches and pain by preventing the blood from pooling. The good news is that most varicose veins will improve within twelve weeks of giving birth. If yours linger, however, there are treatment options, such as surgery, injections, and lasers.

Heredity can make you susceptible to varicose veins, but diet and lifestyle determine if they will develop. Your best dietary protection for healthier veins is to focus on fruits, vegetables, whole grains, and lean sources of protein. Also, eat plenty of foods high in vitamin C, such as citrus, green peppers, and berries, as this vitamin helps to strengthen vein walls.

Supplements that support healthy circulation, such as vitamin C, bioflavonoids, vitamin E, B-complex, and lecithin, can help prevent and treat the road map on your thighs. In addition, beta-carotene supplements improve skin integrity and speed healing of varicose veins.

Great herbal supplements for strengthening veins include horse chestnut and butcher's broom. Horse chestnut contains the active ingredient aescin, which promotes healthy circulation in the veins; it has the added benefit of reducing swelling. Butcher's broom has been found in numerous scientific studies to strengthen veins. Vein-supporting supplements are available as both oral supplements and topical formulas. Many also include nutrients to increase blood flow, such as ginkgo biloba and cayenne.

Spider Veins

Yet another visual reminder of pregnancy, spider veins are thin veins close enough to the surface of the skin that you can see them. Pregnancy tends to bring them out because of the increase in blood volume, as well as hormonal changes. Genetic factors also play a role, so if your mom or sisters have them, you are more likely to as well. The good news is that, unlike varicose veins, spider veins are completely painless. They might disappear after pregnancy or at least fade over time. There are cosmetic treatments (including an injection to make the vein collapse) to get rid of them.

Melasma

I developed melasma, also called the "mask of pregnancy," during my first pregnancy, and it got even worse with my second child. Melasma appears as discolored patches of skin on the face, especially the cheeks, nose, and forehead. An overproduction of melanin, triggered by hormone changes, underlies this condition. Melasma is fairly common and more likely in women with darker skin. For many women, melasma will fade in the months after delivery. However, in others, like me, it can persist. Hydroquinone creams, chemical peels, and topical steroid creams may fade the discolored areas. Make sure to wear a sunscreen with at least SPF 15 every single day, since sun exposure may exacerbate the darkening.

Skin Tags

These are completely normal and harmless and often develop after pregnancy. Skin tags are most likely to form where skin has folds, such as your neck, breasts, and armpits. They don't go away after pregnancy, unfortunately. If your skin tags are irritating (such as one along your bra line) or you just don't like how they look, you can get them removed by a dermatologist, who will cut, freeze, or burn them off.

Moles and Other Marks

Moles have been associated with great beauties, but when does a thing of beauty become life-threatening? Use the ABCDE checklist below to see if you should have a mole checked out:

Asymmetry: One half of the mole does not match the other half.

Border: The border or edges of the mole are ragged, blurred, or irregular.

Color: The color of the mole is not the same throughout or has shades of tan, brown, black, blue, white, or red.

Diameter: The diameter of the mole is larger than the eraser of a pencil.

Evolution: The mole is changing in size, shape, or color.

Cherry hemangiomas comprise another normal, harmless condition, akin to skin tags, that is more common during the aging process and might be slightly more common during pregnancy. These are small red bumps that grow from an enlarged capillary or small vein. If they bother you aesthetically, it is possible to get them removed by a dermatologist.

Cellulite

Cellulite—fatty deposits that cause a dimpled or uneven appearance of the skin on the buttocks and thighs—is all too familiar to many women, especially after childbirth. While the primary treatment is gradual weight loss, anything that increases circulation can help even out puckered skin. The most promising supplements are vitamin C and bioflavonoids, both of which crank circulation into high gear. Also, the herb gotu kola may help iron out the puckers by enhancing connective tissue.

Wrinkles

Is the march of time leaving its mark across your face? As the years pass, and especially after age thirty, collagen and elastin fibers in the skin start to deteriorate. Wrinkles and sagging skin result. The antioxidant nutrients, including vitamin C, vitamin E, beta-carotene, and selenium, may put the brakes on wrinkles, helping skin appear youthful for as long as possible.

The sun's UV rays are perhaps the biggest foe to firm, youthful skin. Frequent or prolonged sun exposure is a major contributor to premature aging and wrinkles. Again, supplementing with antioxidants lessens this source of wrinkles.

Proanthocyanidins are great antioxidants to add to your skin-protecting arsenal. These comprise an antioxidant compound found in many plants, notably pine bark and grape seeds. Proanthocyanidins protect skin collagen (the stuff that makes skin smooth, firm, and strong) from free radical attack and enzymes that would otherwise degrade it. In addition, proanthocyanidins increase blood flow to the skin, so nutrients can be better delivered and waste products shuttled away.

Younger-Looking Skin

Protecting against and reversing UV skin damage goes a long way toward creating youthful-looking skin. Otherwise, UV-generated free radicals result in premature skin aging, such as fine and coarse wrinkling, rough skin texture, dryness, spider veins, and age spots. Topical antioxidants block these UV-induced skin changes and prevent photoaging.[4] The antioxidant vitamin C, for example, has been shown in research to encourage new collagen growth, lighten areas of extra pigmentation, combat inflammation, and even reduce fine lines and wrinkles.[5] Double-blind research in women (in their mid-fifties) shows that a 5 percent alpha-lipoic acid topical cream softens rough skin.[6] And coenzyme Q_{10}, in cream form, has been shown in research to reduce crow's feet around the eyes.[7]

Modern diets contain far lower amounts of silica than in the past, since food processing (particularly of grains) removes much of the silica. Healthy connective tissue, skin, and bones rely on silica: this mineral is needed to form an enzyme, which, in turn, figures in the production of collagen. Supplements of the mineral silica benefit healthy skin (as well as contributing to strong nails and hair), by providing structural integrity to collagen and elastin. Horsetail is a good source of silica.

Silica from foods is converted in the stomach to an active form called orthosilicic acid, which is easily absorbed into the bloodstream through the stomach and intestinal walls. As the years go by, however, stomach acid may not be as strong as it should be, and the conversion of silica to the active form becomes more difficult. Consequently, silica supplements (in the orthosilicic acid form) may be particularly beneficial if you have digestive troubles and would like to improve the look of your skin.

Another option for skin is hyaluronic acid, which is used topically in many face and body creams to hydrate the skin and restore luster and smoothness. It is hydrophilic (water-loving) and helps retain moisture within the skin. Keep in mind: if the weather is dry (or you're in a furnace-heated home), be sure you drink plenty of water when you use a hyaluronic cream; otherwise, it will simply absorb the water already in your system rather than trapping more water in the skin.

A little oil, as it turns out, makes for healthier, younger-looking skin. Both flaxseed and borage oils contain essential fatty acids needed by the body. When a group of women took supplements of flaxseed or borage oil daily for three months, their skin really perked up.[8] Not only did skin circulation improve for these women, they also had less skin irritation and reddening. After just a few weeks of use, women taking borage oil, had 35 percent less skin reddening, and for the flaxseed oil group it lessened by 45 percent; there was no change for the placebo group. The skin of the women taking flaxseed or borage oil even developed a smoother appearance, compared to women taking a placebo.

The omega-3 essential fatty acids EPA and DHA are important for skin, as well. Omega-3s help build strong, vibrant cell membranes, and they also play an important role in calming down inflammation (which helps in cases of acne, eczema, psoriasis, rosacea, and even wrinkles). If you start supplementing with these, you can expect to see a difference in the mirror within a month.

LUXURIOUS HAIR

Just as with skin, the health of your hair is generally a reflection of your internal health. You inherit the color, texture, and even the amount of hair you have, but nutritional choices influence the health, shine, and strength of your hair. Dull, lifeless hair is a sign of a poorly nourished body. Even so, nutrition cannot work miracles (for example, graying hair is not in the realm of nutritional correction).

Why Is Your Hair Falling Out?

Having said all that, though, keep in mind that the shocking amount of hair falling out after you have your baby is normal. Shedding hair in the weeks and months after giving birth is a common occurrence and will not go on forever. I promise: you are not going bald.

Hair undergoes a cyclical process of three phases: growth, rest, and death. During pregnancy, hormones caused an increase to the growing phase of your hair. Thus, your body kept hair strands for longer and they didn't fall out as they would have if you weren't pregnant. With the drop in hormones after delivery, the hairs that were temporarily kept from going into the rest phase now enter that phase and suddenly you are shedding hair all at once. Normal hair growth cycles will resume within six to twelve months after pregnancy.

One note of caution: if your hair loss continues and you have other symptoms (such as depression, feeling cold, constipation), you should talk with your doctor. Thyroid disease can cause hair loss, and this condition can be triggered by pregnancy.

Thinning Hair

Thinning hair is a more common problem for women than men (whereas men are more likely to get a receding hairline). As with men, however, heredity plays a large role in who will develop hair-related disorders. If you are only noticing thinning hair for the first time (and not just the extra shedding in the weeks postpartum), once again the hormonal changes following pregnancy may be to blame. If this is the case, certain herbs that balance hormones (dong quai, ashwagandha, damiana, black cohosh, or sage) could conceivably help, but these herbs should not be used during pregnancy.

Thinning hair may also be triggered by stress, anemia, or thyroid problems. Rapid weight loss from dieting may prompt hair loss as well. While no surefire fixes can reverse thinning hair, you can take some protective steps for the strands you have left. Essential fatty acids (fish, flax, or borage oils), the B vitamin biotin, and silicon are all shown by research to strengthen brittle hair. In addition, zinc promotes hair growth.

And finally, be gentle with your hair so you don't aggravate any loss: avoid blow-drying, curling irons, and perms, as well as any shampoos that contain the ingredients sodium lauryl sulfate, ammonium laureth sulfate, or cocamide DEA because these dry the scalp and hair.

Nutrients for Healthy Hair

The B vitamins are essential for maintaining circulation as well as proper hair growth and color. Vitamins B_6 and B_{12} are important in the formation of red blood cells, which carry oxygen and nutrients to the scalp and hair follicles. Vitamin B_{12} is also crucial in the growth of new hair cells. Pantothenic acid is important for the normal growth and color of hair. A deficiency of biotin may cause hair loss and dry, dull-looking hair. Vitamin C is essential for strong, supple strands of hair that do not break or split. Vitamin C accomplishes this by contributing to healthy sebaceous glands, the oil-producing glands.

Minerals also play their part in lustrous hair. Iron and copper are important in the transport of oxygen to the scalp via the bloodstream. Inadequate amounts of iron may leave the hair and its follicles oxygen-starved, while optimal iron intake and red blood cell levels allow a steady supply of oxygen to reach all tissues, including the scalp and hair. Copper also helps in the formation of hair pigment, while zinc is important in building proteins in the hair and preventing diet-related hair loss.

Choline-stabilized orthosilicic acid was examined in a group of forty-eight women with fine hair who were randomly assigned to take 10 mg of this form of silicon or a placebo daily for nine months.[9] Numerous measurements of hair health showed improvement in this study, including the size of the cross-sectional area of each hair strand, as well as tensile strength, elasticity, and break load, which is how much tugging a strand of hair can take before it snaps. All in all, the women supplementing with silicon for nine months ended up with thicker, healthier hair.

Likewise, another clinical trial found that fifty-five women with thin hair who supplemented with silicon (15 ml as a colloidal silica gel) daily for six months improved their hair thickness by 13 percent.[10] Overall health of the hair, as well as thickness and shine, also improved in this study.

The best-kept secret to a healthy mane of hair may be a simple glass of water. Almost a quarter of the weight of a strand of hair comes from the water locked inside it. This moisture provides suppleness to hair. In addition, the bloodstream is a watery medium that constantly needs replenishing to ensure proper circulation of the nutrients and oxygen needed by the hair and to remove the waste products from the scalp and hair follicles.

TOUGH AS NAILS

As with your hair during pregnancy, you probably noticed that your nails grew faster and stronger during pregnancy. But now that you've had the baby, it may be a different story. Once your hormones settle down, your nails should go back to their normal growth and strength from prepregnancy.

Nails do not readily absorb substances from the environment, which means that creams and lotions applied to the nails are of limited help in addressing brittleness and other issues. Building nail strength through dietary supplements generally has greater success. Nails are composed of keratin, the same protein found in skin and hair. It's not surprising, therefore, that many of the nutrients discussed earlier for glowing skin and vibrant hair also contribute to strong, healthy nails. Keep in mind that a fingernail takes about six months to grow from base to tip, so oral supplements may take months to show an effect.

Nail Nutrients

Low iron levels may lead to weak, thin, flat, or spoon-shaped nails that chip and peel easily. Taking a multivitamin and mineral supplement with iron may correct this problem. Nail strengthening herbs include horsetail and oat straw.

The nutrients that provide the biggest boost to nails are the B-complex vitamins. For instance, by enhancing circulation, vitamins B_6 and B_{12} provide the nail bed with ample amounts of oxygen and nutrients to allow the nails to grow. Inadequate amounts of these B vitamins may result in slow nail growth or weak, easily chipped nails.

One in five people—most of them women—report frail, soft, thin, or brittle nails. The search for a successful treatment for this condition has been elusive. An answer to the problem of brittle nails may be found in veterinary medicine. Animal hooves, which are made from the same protein as human nails, have been shown to benefit from supplementing with the B vitamin biotin. Follow-up studies with humans confirm that biotin supplementation increases nail thickness in a significant number of individuals with brittle nails.

In the study mentioned previously involving fifty women with sun-damaged skin, the researchers also monitored the health of nails and hair over the course of twenty weeks while the women were supplementing with either 10 mg of choline-stabilized orthosilicic acid or a placebo. Comparing the silicon supplementers to those taking a placebo, both nails and hair were found to be significantly less brittle in those taking silicon.

Hangnails, annoying and painful as they are, may be a signal that your diet is low in protein, vitamin C, or folic acid. Boost dietary intake of these nutrients or try supplements.

A BEAUTIFUL MOUTH

Strong, healthy teeth bestow the confidence to flash a broad smile and laugh with an open mouth. Regular brushing and flossing, along with visits to the dentist for periodic cleanings, are necessary to protect your pearly whites. When choosing a toothpaste for your regular brushing, one factor to consider is whether or not to use one with fluoride.

When deciding between toothpastes that contain or omit fluoride, a big part of the decision rests on whether your town's water has naturally high fluoride content or adds fluoride to the water supply. (To find out whether your water contains fluoride, and how much, contact your local water district.) If you're getting fluoride in your water, you don't need toothpaste with even more fluoride.

For sweetening the taste of toothpaste (as well as other dental care products), natural toothpastes often turn to xylitol instead of artificial sweeteners. Xylitol is a naturally occurring sugar substitute that actually makes teeth healthier. Xylitol reduces decay, since plaque-causing bacteria cannot feed on xylitol.

Cavity-free Choppers

Green tea (and to a lesser extent, black and oolong teas) support healthy enamel by making the mouth inhospitable to the bacteria that cause tooth decay. For example, a cross-sectional study of more than six thousand British schoolchildren (fourteen years old) determined that tea-drinking teens experienced fewer cavities than non–tea drinkers. This benefit from tea was not affected by whether or not sugar was added to the tea.[11] Research in animal models confirms the benefit of tea. At the New York University Dental Center, hamsters that consumed water fortified with black tea extract experienced 64 percent fewer cavities.[12]

Neem is derived from the neem tree, which is native to India, where it has been utilized medicinally for so many purposes that it earned the nickname the "village pharmacy." Modern research confirms many of the traditional benefits of neem, including the dental applications, such as a study demonstrating that neem gel works better than chlorhexidine (the active ingredient in certain antiplaque mouthwashes) for lessening plaque.[13] Neem leaf extracts are readily available in toothpaste and other oral hygiene products. Do not use neem during pregnancy, however.

Xylitol is not only found in toothpastes; it's also a sugar alternative in gums and other items. Xylitol reduces sugar intake and has additional dental benefits. Kids who chew xylitol gum have fewer cavities, since xylitol reduces the growth of cavity-causing bacteria.[14]

Additional ways to fight cavities include regular supplementation with the probiotic *Lactobacillus GG* and sucking on vitamin B_6 lozenges.[15]

Gum Disease

Gum disease, or gingivitis, leads to painful, swollen gums; bad breath; and even, potentially, the loss of teeth. The hormones of pregnancy make the teeth more susceptible to plaque development and gingivitis. These problems may continue after pregnancy if you are nursing.

Brushing and flossing frequently, as well as regular cleanings are essential for preventing and treating gum disease. A folic acid mouth rinse (0.1 percent), used twice a day, may lessen the inflammation and bleeding of this condition. Hyaluronic acid, which aids in the repair of connective tissues, improves this condition when applied topically. Taking vitamin C (200–500 mg daily), as well as 60 mg of coenzyme Q_{10} may also help with treatment. Finally, various herbal-based toothpastes or mouthwashes may be of assistance, including bloodroot (sanguinarine), neem, sage, peppermint, chamomile, and myrrh. Although there is no specific research showing a problem with bloodroot or neem during pregnancy or lactation, there is also a lack of data indicating their safety. To err on the side of caution, do not use either of these herbs if you are pregnant or nursing.

Banish Canker Sores

The pain and irritation of canker sores (small ulcers in the lining of the mouth, also called aphthous stomatitis) interfere with pleasurable eating and drinking.

The foaming agent sodium lauryl sulfate (SLS) is a fairly common ingredient in many toothpastes and it does give toothpaste a nice bub-

No Sleep = Gum Disease?

Gum disease progresses more quickly in smokers, which isn't too surprising, but new research shows that not getting enough sleep is the second most telling factor in progressive gum disease. In the study, which tracked a group of workers over a five-year period, 41 percent of those with gum disease were smokers.[17] It seems that sleep shortages impair immune responses, thus allowing the disease to progress more readily. Sleeping seven to eight hours nightly, compared to less than six hours each night, made a big difference in the progression of gum disease. This isn't great news for new parents, but do the best you can to get enough sleep, and, of course, brush and floss regularly.

bly feeling, but the downside is that it's not uncommon for SLS to cause mouth irritation.[16] The most likely reaction to SLS is the development or aggravation of canker sores. If you seem to get a lot of these mouth ulcers, check if your toothpaste contains SLS. If so, it might be prudent to give SLS-free natural toothpastes a try and see if your mouth is happier.

Licorice in the DGL form (deglycyrrhizinated licorice) may be soothing for canker sores. Powdered DGL may be mixed with warm water, swished around the mouth for a few minutes, and then spit out; chewable DGL tablets can also be found. Another topical healer for canker sores is the probiotic *Lactobacillus*, which is available in chewable form. Too little zinc interferes with the body's healing process, so a zinc supplement might help as well.

Sweeter Breath

Bad breath, or halitosis, affects about half the population at one time or another. Simple brushing, flossing, and using a mouthwash rinse goes far toward controlling this problem. Using a tongue scraper may also help quite a bit. Mouthwash containing zinc neutralizes certain sulfur compounds in the mouth associated with bad breath. Herbal mouth rinses (including thyme and eucalyptus extracts) are also powerful agents in combating the bacterial culprits of bad breath.

Smile Brighteners

Many years ago, periodontists (dentists specializing in gum disease) began to recommend that patients brush with a mixture of hydrogen peroxide and baking soda to kill the bacteria that was causing bone loss. After a while, some periodontists realized that this mixture had the side benefit of brightening teeth. Since then, several variations on this tooth-whitening recipe have been developed.

Unfortunately, along with a whiter smile, many teeth-whitening procedures cause tooth sensitivity. In fact, up to half of people aiming for whiter teeth may develop short-term tooth sensitivity. Not surprisingly, then, alternatives for teeth whitening are welcome. Calcium carbonate, bamboo, and silica are natural tooth whiteners that can help erase surface stains in a gentler fashion.

An ounce of prevention goes a long way. Smoking is a no-no for anyone who cares about a bright smile. You should also make sure to rinse and brush after consuming notorious teeth stainers like coffee, tea, grape juice, red wine, and berries. If brushing isn't convenient or accessible, at least chew a stick of natural gum to help buffer against stains.

A FINAL WORD ABOUT NOURISHING YOUR LOOKS

Smooth skin, strong nails, silky hair, and bright teeth are the outward expression of a healthy body. So have fun with luscious-smelling body baths and moisturizers or even paint your nails every color under the sun—but remember that beauty *is* more than skin deep. A healthy body and soul are infinitely more important.

Joy and contentment mean far more at the end of the day than how you look. That's certainly what Heather discovered after becoming a mother: "I cared a lot about my appearance before having my first child, but I actually feel more beautiful now than before parenthood. I stopped bleaching my hair when I got pregnant with my daughter and discovered that I actually have natural highlights. My makeup routine became much more relaxed, and I'm longer embarrassed to go out in public without painting my face. The beauty of becoming a mother made me finally recognize my own natural beauty however 'imperfect' society had taught me it was."

CHAPTER 7

Reconnecting with Passion

No two ways about it: after a baby, your sex life is going to be different. Try to think of it as finding a "new normal" for your sex life—and that shouldn't mean that it's nonexistent. There's the exhaustion, sleep deprivation, new responsibilities—the list goes on and on. Is it any surprise that sex has never been less important to you than it is at this time? Unfortunately, for your husband or partner, sex probably still ranks fairly high on the list of things that interests him. And sex will one day, I promise, matter to you again, too. There are even things you can do to speed along the process to get you to the point that physical intimacy captivates your interest once again.

Sex is one of life's greatest pleasures, and it's an essential part of a fulfilling life—a great sex life helps us feel our best emotionally, mentally, and physically. In the months (or even years) after having a baby, you may be so bone-weary tired that you forget how much fun sex can be. Sometimes it even helps to fake it, at first. "There have been so many times since having children that I thought I wasn't in the mood, but went along with it for my husband's sake. And every single time I've done this I end up really enjoying it and wondering to myself why we don't have sex more often," shares Laura, a mom of two young children.

Before having a baby, you and your lover probably needed nothing more than a glance from each other across a crowded room to set off a chain reaction that ended in sexual fireworks. Nothing quite gets in the way of a sex life like having a new baby in the family. Today you might feel as if it takes nothing less than a nuclear reaction to get things moving in the bedroom. Exciting sex does not have to be relegated to the past; it can be a part of your present and future, too.

ENDING THE DRY SPELL

Most women get the green light from their doctors at the six-week checkup to start having sex again. However, it might be a bit longer for women who have had a Cesarean section. Just because you have the medical okay for physical intimacy doesn't mean that *you* are ready. It's natural for women to lose interest in sex in the weeks (or months) following childbirth. Even after recovering from the physical challenges of the birth process, there's still the 24/7 demands of a newborn and one heck of a hormone roller coaster that often curbs your libido.

Sometimes it seems as if having a child can get in the way—literally—of intimate moments with your husband. "When my daughter was still in our room with us, she fussed and I pulled her over to me to nurse," says new mom Hannah. "A short while later, my husband, who didn't notice any of this, began caressing my back. I thought it was sweet and relaxing, but realized he maybe had more on his mind when he moved his arm around to cup my breast. He was quite surprised to find a baby already there, busy having a snack, which put the kibosh on his plans."

If you're nursing, this adds to the challenge of your flagging libido, since breast-feeding causes estrogen levels to drop. In addition, so many women find their bodies to be under demand all day long that they feel "touched out." And for some women, the physical changes to their bodies leave them feeling unsexy. But remember this: chances are that your husband or partner doesn't care all that much about these postpregnancy changes; he'll just be so happy that you're onboard with the idea of having sex again that stretch marks or extra pounds don't even register with him.

Reasons for Low Sex Drive in New Moms

- **Fluctuating hormones:** Especially if you are still breast-feeding.

- **Exhaustion:** The deepest fatigue you've probably ever had. How do you feel sexy when you can barely keep your head up?

- **Sleep interruptions:** Disrupted sleep every night for months tends to cause stress, moodiness, decreased immune function, and—you guessed it—low sex drive.

- **Body image:** Well, this one I suggest you just get over. Your partner will be so excited that he can have sex, he seriously won't be giving any thought to whether you have a flabby stomach or dark circles under your eyes. Still can't let it go? Then turn out the lights.

- **Discomfort (or fear of it):** If you have a tear, episiotomy, or Cesarean incision that is still healing, you are rightfully cautious about resuming sex. Sex shouldn't hurt after your doc has given you the go-ahead. If it does, get checked for a tear or infection.

- **Lubrication:** Vaginal dryness is a problem in many postpartum women, especially for as long as you're nursing, since low estrogen levels affect vaginal lubrication. Use a lubricant in the meantime. Otherwise, dryness leads to discomfort, which lessens desire—it's a negative feedback loop.

RECONNECTING WITH YOUR PARTNER

Finding your sexual self again after having a baby is not just about reconnecting with your passion; it's also about reconnecting with your partner. In the process of restoring or strengthening your intimacy, passion for each other should naturally follow. Indeed, it becomes a circle in which greater intimacy leads to more and better sex, the sex, in turn, primes the feelings of intimacy, and so on. And don't underestimate the value of a door lock! Once your kids become mobile, it's essential. "Locking the bedroom door allows me to relax and not worry that someone will burst into the room unexpectedly," notes Megan, mom of two preschoolers.

As you navigate this postbaby time in your relationship, it is more important than ever to recognize that men and women approach sex very differently. A man's body responds more quickly to sexual cues. Compounding this difference, many men feel desired and loved as a result of having sexual contact, while most women need to feel intimacy and emotional connection *before* their sexual desire kicks into high gear. This male/female mismatch has been at the root of many couples' downfall. Working together to find a balance that is fulfilling to both partners is vital to a relationship's success. If you're a new dad reading this chapter and looking for tips to get your partner in the mood, then pay attention: walking the halls with a cranky baby should be your new go-to foreplay for the next few months. A mom who gets a bit more sleep is much more likely to respond to a suggestion of sex.

"Make time for your relationship." This is advice most new moms hear. But frankly, if you don't have time to shower, it's pretty challenging to find time for a candlelit dinner. One of the most important things to remember is that these superbusy and sleep-deprived months of having a new infant are not going to last forever. Once things settle down a bit after the newborn period, take the time to nourish your physical connection with your husband or partner.

In the meantime, even if physical intimacy feels impossible, you can still find ways to connect emotionally. For example, Amanda shares that once she and her husband got a sitter so they could go shopping at the new Ikea in town. "Instead of just checking off items on our shopping list, we brought some red wine (in a coffee travel mug) and leisurely explored the store hand in hand. We've had similar 'dates' at Costco," she adds. "With the right attitude, an errand can turn into a fun, bonding experience."

NATURAL RELATIONSHIP STAGES

Couples in a long-term relationship need to keep their expectations realistic. As fun and exhilarating as it is to fall in love, this level of excitement is not possible to maintain. This initial infatuation stage—when a couple thinks of nothing but each other and the sex is thrilling and frequent—is not going to last forever. As a relationship stabilizes, it moves into a phase of emotional attachment, where real love blooms. This represents a deeper level of commitment and also allows you to incorporate the sexual relationship into the rest of your life; sex is no longer all-consuming.

Some couples mourn the loss of the infatuation stage, and this may lead to couple trouble. However, the most successful long-term relationships are the ones that nurture and maintain the attachment phase. These couples recognize that moving out of infatuation and into attachment does not mean falling out of love; it simply means that the relationship has matured. But by no means does this mean that sex can't still be great after many years of marriage and the addition of kids. In fact, as Andrea confides: "Now that our kids are in preschool, I'm thrilled to discover that my sex life with my husband has not only

Green Light for Postbaby Sex

For a vaginal birth, most OBs okay intercourse six weeks after birth. Why the wait (besides the fact that you are so tired and consumed with the baby that sex is the furthest thing from your mind)? The medical reason is this: the cervix needs to close completely to prevent the risk of infection and, of course, the vaginal tissues need a bit of time to heal. Honor your own timetable. Just because you have the medical green light from your doctor at six weeks doesn't mean that's a mandate. If you still have pain and soreness, give yourself some more time to heal.

For C-section moms, it will take a bit longer so you don't tear the internal sutures that hold the abdominal muscles together. A good sign that you're healed enough to consider sex is if you can push on the scar without pain.

And when you do start having sex again, don't forget birth control! Nursing is not a foolproof form of birth control. Just ask my mom (her second child was born a mere eleven months after the first—whoops).

recovered, it's the best ever. So my message to other moms would be this: don't give up!"

COUPLE TROUBLE

Relationship difficulties, such as emotional issues and rejection by a partner, are fingered as the reason for failed marriages by 40 percent of women and 43 percent of men. Sexual difficulties usually go hand in hand with these problems. Many postbaby marriages begin to morph into a business partnership of sorts, where housekeeping, finances, and social obligations shove intimacy to the back of the line. Poor communication, anger, a lack of trust, and a lack of connection are invariably factors here. These issues must be dealt with before sexual connection can be restored. If a couple has drifted so far apart that they cannot find their way back to intimacy on their own, a couples counselor may help.

If a couple's relationship problems seem relatively minor, the fixes might also be minor. For example, some couples keep the spark alive by making dates with each other to refocus some energy on intimacy. Spending time together, with no other distractions, may rekindle a spark.

THE 'RIGHT' AMOUNT OF SEX

Many people wonder how often "normal" couples have sex. The short answer is that there is no normal or right amount of sex. How much sex is right for a particular couple is determined by many factors and changes over the course of a relationship. There is certainly more sex at the "honeymoon" stage. Other factors include the sexual clock of each partner, how busy they are, how many distractions they face (such as multiple jobs, conflicting job shifts, small children at home, and so on), and the aging process. There is wide variation, but the average for couples in their twenties is about twice a week, versus an average of twice a month for couples in their sixties (assuming an absence of sexual dysfunction).

But there is no reason for you to feel that you have to match any average. If you're happy having daily sex or once-a-year sex, then there is no problem. Problems only arise when one or both of you are not content with the frequency.

GET IN TOUCH

Of all the senses, touch contributes the most directly to sexual pleasure. Touch stimulates the release of oxytocin, one of the pleasure hormones. Oxytocin reaches peak levels at the point of orgasm, but it contributes to a feeling of being bonded with your partner as well. Oxytocin is also released during the gentle touching of massage, hugging, and kissing. As you probably also know from all the baby books you've read in the past few months, oxytocin is secreted when you nurse your baby, too.

After a baby arrives, many couples stop holding hands and may no longer touch at all in any affectionate ways, other than intercourse (and even that might be on hiatus!). All too often, a new mother may end up feeling as though any touch that her partner initiates is simply a come-on to sex. Touching each other—an arm around a shoulder, a hand resting on a thigh—at times that do not lead to sexual encounters helps build an overall closeness that leads to more intimacy and better sex.

THE SCENT OF LOVE

Scents have been recognized by every culture as aphrodisiacs. Fragrances are integral to seduction, fertility rites, and marriage ceremonies in most cultures. Today's world, with its booming perfume and cologne businesses, is no exception. Explore the array of scents through scented candles, potpourri, incense, perfume, cologne, and/or scented massage oil.

Sexual attraction is also affected by smells we don't even realize are there, called pheromones. Many sexual aspects of the lives of other animals are governed by pheromones, and humans are not so different. In a pair of studies, one conducted with women and the other with men, synthesized pheromones were applied daily and sexual behaviors were tracked for a few months. In both studies, the men and women wearing pheromones noted significantly more sexual encounters (intercourse, kissing, petting, affection, and dates) than men and women given a fake spray. Clearly, pheromones attract the opposite sex.

So, new dads: you might want to stack the odds in your favor and try to perk up some interest in your sleep-deprived, frazzled wife, but I wouldn't necessarily count on pheromones sparking enough sexual interest if sleep is still being interrupted by a baby every night. Desire for sleep generally trumps desire for sex.

SETTING THE MOOD

Food and sex often share an intimate bond. But besides the individual foods with reputations as aphrodisiacs, food in general often plays a big role during the seduction or courtship stage of a relationship. And it doesn't need to end there. Romantic dinners may continue to be a prelude to an evening of great sex. For many years after becoming parents, Laura and her husband celebrated every Valentine's Day by ordering takeout and setting up the table for a romantic meal, either when the kids were asleep or while they were watching a DVD. Even with small kids in the house, there are still ways to celebrate romantic holidays.

Setting a romantic mood often starts with selecting great music for the background. Music may ease the transition from a hectic day to an amorous evening by helping to relax and soothe the body. Many couples have certain types of music or individual songs that serve as cues that a romantic tryst is forthcoming. So switch the Laurie Berkner playlist for Josh Groban instead. It may help get your mind out of "mommy mode."

TALKING OPENLY

For both women and men, talking about sex in a personal way may be a scary endeavor—but it comes with great rewards. Sharing your sexual needs, desires, and wishes with your partner is much more effective than hoping that your partner is a mind reader. Before you start such an important conversation, it is a good idea to spend some time beforehand organizing your thoughts. Next, make sure that your partner is in the mood to have such a talk; if he or she is distracted or tired, it's best to reschedule. Most important of all, make sure you emphasize the positive side of your sex life and relationship so that the conversation doesn't backfire. For example, instead of saying, "I just don't want to have sex anymore since I'm so busy with the new baby, so stop asking!" try "I might need a little time to adjust to being a parent. Can you understand that I might not feel supersexy for a while?"

Being open and creative helps in other ways, as well. Naptime or while the kids are watching a DVD may be a great time to fit in some intimacy during the day (since the kids are asleep during naptime and preoccupied while watching a DVD). And, as cosleeping mom Heather points out, "We take full advantage of having a large house to find creative times and places to be intimate!"

KEGEL MAGIC

Engaging in exercise of any kind generally contributes to a better sex life, but a special type of exercise called Kegels may specifically improve sexual performance. Kegels focus on improving the muscle tone of a set of muscles in the genital region that rarely get attention otherwise. Kegel exercises were developed in the 1950s by a surgeon named Arnold Kegel with the goal of restoring or improving the tone of the pubococcygeal muscles, otherwise known as the pelvic floor. The pelvic floor often gets weaker during pregnancy and childbirth (as well as during the older years, as a result of the aging process).

To perform Kegel exercises, you squeeze together the muscles of the pelvic floor, as if you were trying to stop urine in midstream. Squeeze and release in sets of ten several times a day. This should strengthen muscle tone. Kegels are recommended for some women to prevent incontinence, but another benefit is improved sexual pleasure in many women.

HOW FATIGUE AND DEPRESSION SAP SEXUAL ENERGY

Since your baby was born, how often has fatigue prevented you or your partner from engaging in a bedtime romp? Yep, that's what I thought. Fatigue is the number-one killer of the new parent's sex life. Life with a new baby is so packed that sex is simply crowded out of the day (or week, or even month).

Although eight hours of shut-eye is the standard recommendation, almost half of average Americans sleep only six hours or less each night. Of course, new parents are likely to be getting far less sleep than that! Sleep deprivation saps your interest in many activities, including sex. Furthermore, lack of sleep is linked to depressed mood and crankiness, two qualities that don't dovetail with high sexual interest, pleasure, and performance.

Being "in the mood" is a whole lot less likely if you're in a bad mood. This is common sense, but if you doubt it, a handful of studies have measured sexual response during positive and negative moods. No big surprises here: being in a good mood is more conducive to feeling sexually aroused.

In their extreme form, mood problems may end up as full-blown depression. Depression may be caused by a chemical imbalance in the brain, severe stress, grief, emotional conflict, or a combination of these factors. Depression is widespread, especially among women. Twice as many women as men suffer from depression, with about 20 percent of women developing depression some time in their lives.

Depression will certainly put a serious damper on sexual desire—as well as many other aspects of life—and it needs to be treated before learning whether there are other causes of the sexual dysfunction. In many cases, resolving the depression takes care of the sexual problem. Ironically, many antidepressant medications have sexual side effects.

WOMEN'S SEXUAL CONCERNS

Women's sexual problems have not gotten the attention from the medical community that they merit. Unlike men—who, if they can't get an erection, simply can't have intercourse—women who are not sexually responsive can still have sex. It's just no fun.

Over the years, many women brave enough to share their sexual frustrations with their doctors were merely told to use a lubricant. Or worse, their sexual health concerns were dismissed as either psychological or emotional problems. While the sexual problems of women (like those of men) are usually physical in nature, these physical causes can be treated. Thankfully, in recent years the medical community has begun paying much more attention to this issue. If your lack of interest in sex is not just a temporary setback because of a new baby in the house, talk to your doctor. Loss of desire and other sexual problems are much more common in women than you might think, but it doesn't need to be this way. Most of these problems are treatable.

Four Types of Female Sexual Dysfunction

The first category of female sexual dysfunction is known as low sexual desire. In this case, a woman simply has a lack of interest in sex. Depression is a common cause of dampened libido. Certain medications may also be to blame.

Second is sexual arousal disorder. In such cases, a woman lacks adequate vaginal lubrication and accompanying swelling of the external genitalia. Other aspects of arousal, such as nipple sensitivity, increased clitoral and labial sensation, and vaginal dilation, are generally impaired, as well. Female arousal, like male arousal, requires well-functioning circulation and nerve fibers. Smoking and cardiovascular disease are culprits here. If the problem is primarily inadequate lubrication for comfortable sex, use of topical lubricants may help.

The third category of problems facing women is difficulty in reaching orgasm or the inability to achieve orgasm. Some women have never had an orgasm, while others used to have orgasms, but after surgery, trauma, medication use, or hormone deficiency no longer have them. Since most women reach orgasm as a result of clitoral stimulation (as opposed to just vaginal penetration)—and the clitoris is not directly stimulated during intercourse—the problem might easily be solved by providing the right type of stimulation (manual, oral, or with a vibrator directly to the clitoris). Before a woman assumes she has an orgasm disorder, she first should determine whether or not clitoral stimulation results in orgasm. If so, then the problem may be solved simply by changing sexual technique.

The final category is sexual pain disorders. When intercourse is painful, a woman is said to suffer from dyspareunia. Numerous factors may account for this common problem. In one survey, 18 percent of healthy women reported experiencing frequent pain during intercourse. If the pain is at the vaginal entrance, the problem might be related to a local irritation as a result of spermicides or a yeast infection. Pain deeper in the vagina is commonly caused by the penis being inserted before the woman is fully aroused, which means that the vagina has not yet had a chance to expand. Endometriosis and fibroid tumors also account for some cases of dyspareunia.

In some women, the pain is related to a condition called vaginismus, in which the lower third of the vagina has recurrent involuntary spasms. These spasms interfere with or even prevent intercourse. This is much less common than the other female sexual dysfunctions discussed in this section and is often triggered by past sexual trauma, such as sexual abuse or painful intercourse that, in turn, causes spasms in anticipation that future intercourse might also be painful. Vaginismus is generally treated with a two-pronged approach of psychological counseling and a procedure in which the woman uses a series of graduated dilators while focusing on the different sensations of muscle relaxation and contraction.

IS YOUR PROBLEM IN YOUR MEDICINE CHEST?

Drugs, both prescription and over the counter, can have a big impact on sexual health. They can interfere with blood flow to the genitals, contribute to vaginal dryness, dampen libido, and alter hormones involved in the sexual response. It is important to consult a physician to rule these out as the source of any sexual problems. Many people have discovered that they traded in one health problem for another with a new medication—that is, their initial health complaint was resolved but now they face sexual dysfunction. There may be drug or treatment alternatives that treat the initial problem without the specter of sexual side effects.

Many drugs chemically crush the libido. While there are alternatives that you can explore, remember that your health comes first. Don't discontinue a medication without discussing it with your health care provider first. If medications you need are potentially causing sexual dissatisfaction, talk to your doctor about switching to another medication or changing the dose of your existing prescription.

The most common medications that cause sexual side effects are certain types of antidepressants, high blood pressure medications, antacids, and appetite suppressants.

APHRODISIAC HERBS AND SUPPLEMENTS

The search for aphrodisiacs dates back millennia. Aphrodisiacs—named for Aphrodite, the Greek goddess of love and beauty—work in many different ways. Some are tonics that crank up vitality; others more directly affect the reproductive system. And the most highly prized aphrodisiacs of all have a direct sparking effect on the libido, stirring desire and even improving performance and pleasure.

If your libido has gone missing and you're ready to coax your mojo back, check out these herbal sex boosters. The vitamins, minerals, amino acids, and herbs described below have documented aphrodisiac abilities—just don't use them all at the same time. Be selective and choose the one or two that seem best suited to your situation. If those don't seem to work for you, move on and try a new one.

Note: There are many herbs and dietary supplements to help men overcome impotence and boost male desire. They won't be included here since most husbands are so sexually deprived at this point that that's rarely an issue for them.

Arginine

The amino acid arginine has been tested for its ability to enhance arousal for both men and women. Arginine is found in protein-rich foods, such as soy, brown rice, chicken, dairy products, and nuts. It is also available as a dietary supplement.

Arginine raises levels of nitric oxide in the blood and body tissues. This, in turn, increases the blood flow that is necessary for sexual arousal. When researchers compared arginine (given in combination with ginkgo, ginseng, damiana, and fourteen other vitamins and minerals) to a placebo in women lacking sexual desire, 62 percent of the arginine group reported significant improvement in their sexual satisfaction, compared to only 38 percent of the placebo group[1] Similarly, 64 percent of the arginine group reported a boost in sexual desire.

Damiana

Damiana is a time-honored aphrodisiac herb, long used by herbalists in Mexico to improve sexual interest and response. Traditionally, damiana has been recommended for women, although more recent animal research shows a sexual pick-me-up in both men and women.[2] There have been a few studies with a combination herbal formula (based on damiana, as well as ginseng and ginkgo) indicating successful results in women. Although there is no research showing damiana to be harmful during pregnancy, because this herb was used traditionally to cause miscarriage, it is best to avoid using it during pregnancy.

Dong Quai

Dong quai (also called Chinese angelica) is often referred to as the "female ginseng." Traditionally, dong quai is believed to have a balancing, or adaptogenic, effect on the female hormonal system, acting as an all-purpose sexual and reproductive tonic. It has a long history of use in both Europe and Asia. In fact, it has been used in China for more than two thousand years as a stimulant for women's reproductive systems. This herb should not be used during pregnancy or while breastfeeding, due to a paucity of safety data.

Epimedium

Epimedium (also known as horny goat weed) is considered an aphrodisiac or sexual tonic. It has a two-thousand-year history of use in

Traditional Chinese Medicine. Legend has it that this aptly named herb gained its moniker when a goat herder noted the randy behavior of goats after they ate from a particular patch of weeds. Epimedium stimulates sensory nerves that have an indirect effect on increasing sexual desire.

Ginkgo

The herb ginkgo is no Johnny-come-lately. This species is at least 200 million years old, and individual trees can live for hundreds of years. As far back as 2800 BCE, ginkgo was reported to have a medicinal effect in the Chinese *Materia Medica* (an herbal encyclopedia). In ancient times, the root and kernel of the fruit were used to nourish sexual vitality.

Only in the past few decades have the leaves of the ginkgo tree become the focus of natural medicine. An extract from these leaves has been widely studied for its ability to boost blood flow all over the body, particularly blood flow in the brain, which is thought to enhance cognitive health. But just as ginkgo keeps the blood vessels flowing to the brain healthy, it also promotes healthy blood flow throughout the body, including the genitals in both men and women. There are anecdotal reports and some limited research involving individuals with antidepressant-induced low sex drive recovering when supplementing with ginkgo. Do not take ginkgo if you're pregnant or nursing, due to lingering doubts about the safety of this herb during those times.

Ginseng

Ginseng is another long-respected herb, with a five-thousand-year-old reputation in China as a cure-all. Ginseng root was so highly prized in ancient China that only emperors could collect the herb. Similarly, Ottoman Empire sultans boosted their sexual potency with ginseng. Current scientific evidence about the sexual powers of this herb for men suggests that the old stories might have something to them. However, men are not the only ones to benefit from ginseng. According to a new study conducted in Korea, women taking ginseng felt more easily aroused in the bedroom and reported overall improvements in their sex lives.[3]

There are three types of ginseng: Asian, Siberian, and American. The most commonly used ginseng type is Asian ginseng, often labeled as Panax, Chinese, or Korean ginseng. American ginseng is closely related to Asian ginseng. Siberian ginseng, also called eleuthero, is not as closely related to the other two herbs, but generally has similar effects. Ginseng should not be taken during pregnancy because there are some animal studies linking this herb to the potential for birth defects. Nursing women should also avoid it due to a lack of safety data.

Maca

Maca, a root from the Peruvian Andes, has potent libido-enhancing power. Although it has only recently gained popularity in the United States, it's been used in Peru for thousands of years. Traditionally, Peruvians relied on this herb to boost energy and fertility. Today, research demonstrates that this herb increases desire and sexual function in both men and women.[4]

Mucuna Pruriens

Mucuna pruriens (also known as velvet bean) is an herb indigenous to India. The Ayurvedic tradition classifies this herb as an aphrodisiac. Mucuna pruriens has been shown to increase testosterone levels, which could contribute to a libido-boosting effect. Additional research in humans is warranted, and to be safe (at least until there is research showing safety), do not use this herb during pregnancy or lactation.

Muira Puama

Muira puama, an herb derived from an Amazonian tree, has some documentation as a sexual enhancer. In one study with 202 women reporting low sex drive, a combination of Muira puama and ginkgo resulted in significant improvements in terms of desire, intercourse, and satisfaction with sex life.[5] Due to a lack of safety data, it is wise not to use this herb during pregnancy or lactation.

Rhodiola

Rhodiola, an herb that also sometimes goes by the name golden root, has been used traditionally in Russia for energy. Research (both in Russia and in the United States) indicates that rhodiola improves cognitive function and provides a mood lift by boosting production of serotonin in the brain. There are early reports of improved sexual satisfaction with this herb as well.

Vitex

Vitex also goes by the name chasteberry, since it was at one time believed to quell sexual desire. Modern herbalists, however, believe that vitex does not result in chastity, but rather corrects hormone imbalances. In essence, vitex is thought to balance sexual energy, to either decrease or increase it, as needed. Vitex may take several months to show an effect; however, it should be immediately discontinued if a woman becomes pregnant, since there is a slight concern that this herb (by encouraging menstruation) could interfere with pregnancy.

PILLOW TALK

A fulfilling sex life takes more than just popping an aphrodisiac herb or a dietary supplement. Great sex takes intimacy, communication, good dietary choices, a healthy lifestyle, time, and energy. It's common sense: if something is good for your overall health, well-being, and relationship, then it is most likely good for your sex life, too.

CHAPTER 8

Fighting Fatigue

When you were pregnant, veteran moms probably warned you about the sleep deprivation ahead, but there just isn't any way to understand how tired you'll actually be until your baby arrives. And how tired will you be? More tired than you have ever been before and more tired than you thought it was possible for a person to be and continue to function. I remember one time, after my second child was born, I was driving and I actually forgot how to turn on the windshield wipers in my car. That was a day I put the laundry and other chores aside and made sure to nap while the little ones were napping.

This isn't a chapter purporting to offer the secret answer to getting your baby to sleep through the night. Rather, it will share information on how to make the most of what little rest time you have and tips about how to eat or supplement your way to alertness when more sleep just isn't an option.

SLEEP ISN'T A LUXURY

Our culture treats sleep like a luxury, but there's no escaping the biological necessity of sleep. Most people need seven to eight hours a night to function optimally. Well, that's just not going to happen for most parents of very young children. Being shortchanged even just two hours of sleep nightly (that is, snoozing for six hours) dings your thinking ability. In fact, research shows that sleeping only six hours each night for numerous days in a row results in cognitive deficits equivalent to people who have stayed awake for thirty-six hours or more nonstop.

Even so, somehow parents keep functioning on too little sleep because, well, you do what you have to do. It's amusing that it may even take an adjustment period to begin sleeping again. Melissa recalls that she had more than three years of not having a single night of uninterrupted sleep: "I had two kids pretty close together in age. My first child started sleeping through the night just as pregnancy insomnia set in during the end of my second pregnancy. I remember the first night my second child slept all night (which meant that I slept through the night for the first time in three years), I woke up with a terrible crick in my neck and thought to myself, 'Wow, I guess I am out of practice and need to ease back into this sleep business!' "

YOUR ENERGY PATTERNS

Most people have cyclical energy patterns that naturally ebb and flow. Perhaps you're a morning person and get more done by 9 a.m. than some people do all day. Or perhaps, as the sun goes down, you just start to get charged up. You may be a zombie until you've had your morning coffee. Or maybe you're worthless for the two hours after lunch. Each of us has our own energy rhythm.

It's valuable to discover the natural rhythms of your personal energy cycles and work with them, instead of against them, as much as your schedule will allow. Try keeping a record of your activities for a week or two, noting which times of day are consistently high-, medium-, and low-energy times for you. Then utilize your energy peaks for plowing through your workload, and try to match your energy valleys with times you can relax and recharge.

THE BEST SLEEP ARRANGEMENT FOR YOUR FAMILY

Where should everyone in a family sleep? Wherever gets everyone in the house the most sleep is the answer I believe in, whether that's a crib in a separate bedroom, a bassinet in the parents' room, or cosleeping in a family bed, where everyone is together. Cosleeping isn't for everyone, but many families find that a family bed gets them more snooze-time overall. Others, however, find that having a baby in bed with them interferes with sleep. There is no right or wrong answer.

Jen, a mom of twins, found that she and her husband slept much better when they brought their babies in bed with them, but only after switching to a king-size bed. "When we had a queen and four people in it, my husband and I woke up with backaches every morning!" she recalls. Jen found that knowing her babies were close and safe let her relax and sleep more deeply, and it certainly helped with the logistics of breast-feeding two babies.

Cosleeping families are starting to come out of the closet, thanks, in part, to the support of a slew of modern baby experts supportive of this sleep style. Even Dr. Richard Ferber—the pediatrician whose name became shorthand for solitary infant sleep—regrets his earlier anti–family-bed stance. Many (but not all!) families find that everyone tends to get more sleep in a family bed.

The latest research on cosleeping completely overturns the myths about the family bed, finding that babies who share sleep with parents are happier, throw fewer tantrums, exhibit fewer emotional and behavioral

Cosleeping Safety Rules

If you are going to cosleep, it's important to follow safe-sleep guidelines:

- Don't smoke in bed.
- Don't use alcohol or drugs that lead to grogginess.
- Put the baby on mom's side, rather than in the middle.
- Use a firm mattress.
- Eliminate crevices at the head and foot of the bed.
- Keep your pillow away from the baby.

problems, and are less susceptible to peer pressure later in life. There's practically no scientific evidence to support any benefit of solitary infant sleep, particularly in matters of independence. In fact, there is research to the contrary, indicating that solitary sleepers are less independent.

Cosleeping is not an all-or-nothing proposition. As new mom Veronica shares: "I have just learned that we all sleep better if my six-month-old daughter starts the night in her crib, but comes in with us later in the night when she wakes up to nurse." Going with the flow helps maximize sleep.

FOODS AND DRINKS FOR AN ENERGETIC DAY

It's bad enough that your teething infant kept you up half the night—now is not the time to feed your fatigue with poor food choices. When your baby seems intent on sabotaging your nighttime hours, it's more important than ever to nourish your energy stores during the day.

Breakfast

Now that you are a mother yourself, you're going to find that your own mom sure was right about a lot of things (I certainly found this to be true!). So here's one more thing your mother knew best: breakfast *is* the most important meal of the day. Skipping breakfast is a surefire way to zap your vim and vigor. Research has found that breakfast skippers struggle with more weight problems and low energy levels later in the day than people who take the time to eat breakfast. Even if you "catch up" by eating a well-balanced lunch, you will never regain the energy you would have had by taking ten minutes to eat a nutritious breakfast.

Here's part of the problem: people who skip breakfast in order to cut calories often snack more later in the day and overeat at evening meals, which, ironically, results in a greater struggle with weight problems and chronic low energy levels. By contrast, eating breakfast boosts energy levels all day and helps you maintain a healthy weight.

The basics for an energy-boosting breakfast are simple:

1. Make it light by avoiding sugar and too much fat.

2. Go easy on the coffee and other caffeinated beverages.

3. Choose foods with a mix of protein and carbohydrates.

Examples of fast, easy breakfasts that fit these rules include yogurt and granola, toast and a hard-boiled egg, or cereal with milk.

Lunchtime

Just as breakfast helps you start the day right, what and how much you eat for lunch sets the tone for the rest of the day. Revitalizing lunches will follow these energy-boosting rules:

1. Eat lunch in moderation. Too few calories leave you hungry and lacking stamina for the afternoon, but too many calories may leave you fit for nothing more strenuous than an afternoon nap. The happy medium is a light meal of five hundred calories that will refuel your energy without leading to drowsiness.

2. Fatty meals trigger feelings of tiredness by increasing levels of chemicals that lower your fatigue threshold. Low-fat lunches are a prime component of a get-things-done afternoon.

3. Balance your carbs and protein. An all-carbohydrate lunch, such as pasta with marinara sauce, raises levels of a brain chemical called serotonin, which, in turn, makes you drowsy. By contrast, protein triggers the release of norepinephrine, a brain chemical that helps boost energy and mood. So an energizing lunch will contain a mix of carbohydrates and protein, such as a bean-and-cheese burrito with rice, to maximize the fuel from carbohydrates while getting the energy lift from protein.

Snack Defensively

Making frequent stops to refuel throughout the day is a great way to sustain energy levels (especially if you're nursing); that is, if you choose the right snacks.

Sugary treats may provide a quick fix to lagging energy levels, but you'll be setting yourself up for an inevitable crash. Sugar from cookies, candy, and soda pop is dumped into the bloodstream, causing a dramatic rise in blood sugar. The immediate response from the pancreas is to counteract the sugar spike with the hormone insulin, which hustles excess sugar from the blood into the cells. Blood sugar levels then plummet; often to even lower levels than before you consumed the sugary snack!

Studies show that individuals who frequent the candy aisle undermine their energy levels in another way—by consuming inadequate amounts of the energizing nutrients vitamin C, the B vitamins, magnesium, potassium, and zinc.

The best snacks are readily available, take little time to prepare, and taste great. For example, bagels with a high-protein spread, fat-free crackers and cheese, fresh fruit and cottage cheese, or low-fat tortilla chips and bean dip are all great mini-meals that help feed your energy needs—not your fatigue.

Drink water or noncaffeinated beverages with every snack (again, especially if you are nursing). Mild dehydration is a common but often neglected source of fatigue. And since thirst is a poor indicator of fluid needs, a good rule of thumb is to drink twice as much as it takes to quench your thirst.

CAFFEINE: A DOUBLE-EDGED SWORD

If more sleep is out of the question but you simply must be alert, then coffee, tea, and caffeinated soda all provide a hit of caffeine, a proven way to banish fatigue, at least for a few hours. If you find yourself turning to caffeine to get through the day, you're not alone. More than 80 percent of Americans consume at least some caffeine every day.

Use this pick-me-up judiciously, however: at a moderate intake, coffee and other caffeine sources help people think faster, concentrate better, stay alert, and work more efficiently, but when intake creeps above one or two cups a day, this energy booster turns into an energy sapper. A vicious cycle may result, in which you drink more coffee to avoid fatigue and other withdrawal symptoms.

Who knew that coffee—once viewed as an indulgent vice—might

actually be a disease-fighter in a "to go" cup? Scientists have recently uncovered healthy links between coffee and a lower risk of diabetes, Parkinson's disease, colon cancer, cirrhosis of the liver, and gallstones. Need even more reasons to pour yourself a steaming mug? Coffee lifts your mood, relieves headaches, and even keeps cavities at bay. And in the largest, longest-running study to date, researchers found that—looking at overall death rates—coffee drinkers may even live a little longer than those who don't drink coffee.[1]

While pregnant women should continue to limit caffeine to the amount in about one cup of coffee (200 mg), due to concerns about miscarriage, worries about breast cancer and caffeine appear to be unfounded. After studying more than 85,000 women for more than two decades, Harvard researchers concluded that coffee and tea do not increase the risk of breast cancer.[2] Phew! The role of caffeine in fibrocystic breast disease, however, remains controversial. Some women find that removing caffeine from their diets resolves breast symptoms brought on by this condition.

The main downside from caffeine seems to be the insomnia, irritability, anxiety, increased urination, diarrhea, and/or heartburn that it may trigger in either caffeine-sensitive people ingesting small amounts or other people consuming large amounts of caffeine (say, more than three cups of coffee). In addition, anyone at increased risk for osteoporosis may still want to limit coffee intake. And, of course, regular caffeine users will develop a dependence, with withdrawal symptoms (namely, headache, nervousness, and nausea) developing if more than twenty-four hours goes by without caffeine.

HERBAL ENERGIZERS

While nothing but sleep itself will repay your sleep debt, in a pinch you can turn to energizing herbs and supplements to perk up.

Start your search for natural energy support by checking the basics. How's your core nutrition? Numerous nutritional surveys report the same dismal news: many Americans walk around with marginal deficiencies of a number of basic vitamins and minerals. Since almost every vitamin and mineral plays a part in the complex process that turns food and oxygen into energy, even a marginal deficiency may lead to lethargy. A high-potency daily multivitamin/mineral supplement covers the bases, but make sure that it contains the key players in energy production: vitamin C, magnesium, and B-complex vitamins.

Iron deficiency is an all-too-frequent cause of chronic weariness, particularly in women. Although only a small percentage of women are anemic (the final stage of iron deficiency), almost 40 percent of younger women have low iron stores and twice this number of exercising women are deficient in this important mineral. Iron deficiency leads to fatigue, as the brain and muscles are literally starved of energy-giving oxygen. It might be worth a quick check for anemia at your doctor's office. If so, your doctor will work with you to determine how much iron you should take as a supplement.

Green foods, such as the micro-algaes spirulina, chlorella, and Klamath Lake blue-green algae—as well as cereal grasses, such as barley grass and wheat grass—are chock-full of vitamins, minerals, amino acids, and essential fatty acids. These green "superfoods" provide concentrated nutrition to boost lagging energy. Green foods earn their moniker through the green-colored substance they all contain: chlorophyll. The chemical structure of chlorophyll is nearly identical to hemoglobin (the red, oxygen-transporting pigment in human blood).

Bee products might deserve their buzz. Both bee pollen supplements and royal jelly increase energy levels. Worker bees produce royal jelly (a nutritious, creamy-white substance) as a special food for the queen bee alone. Because they consume this royal jelly, queen bees live for years—remarkable considering that the worker bees live for only a matter of weeks. Traditionally, royal jelly's been taken for its rejuvenating properties, and research in animal models confirms that this bee product improves energy levels.

Coenzyme Q_{10} is a vitaminlike substance that helps in the complicated process of converting food into energy; it's naturally concentrated in the mitochondria of cells, which are the powerhouses of energy production. Most coenzyme Q_{10} is synthesized by the body in a complex process that converts the amino acid tyrosine into coenzyme Q_{10}, with the help of eight vitamins and several trace minerals. Coenzyme Q_{10} can boost vitality in generally healthy people, especially after age forty, when endogenous coenzyme Q_{10} production starts to peter out.

Yet another potentially invigorating supplement, alpha-lipoic acid, is also needed by the body during the process of burning food for energy. Alpha-lipoic acid supplements increase mitochondrial energy production, giving the body a lift.

Several herbs support healthy energy levels by nourishing the adrenal glands and, in turn, the important connections between the hypothalamus, the pituitary gland, and the adrenal glands (known as the hypothalamus-pituitary-adrenal axis). Ginseng and licorice are two herbs that support a healthy adrenal gland, and in this way shore up energy levels. (Ginseng is best avoided during pregnancy because of preliminary animal research linking it to an increased risk of birth defects, and licorice should not be used due to a risk of miscarriage or early delivery. The safety of neither of these herbs has been established during nursing, so they should also be avoided by breast-feeding mothers.) Similarly, the Chinese herb schisandra has been found to reduce fatigue. Ginkgo, which works by increasing blood flow to the brain and boosting mental alertness, is a welcome energy booster; gotu kola also stimulates the brain; and other herbs, such as green tea, guarana, and kola nut, provide energy through their caffeine content. Do not take ginkgo if you're pregnant or nursing, since its safety has yet to be confirmed by scientific studies.

INSOMNIA IS UNFAIR

How's this for unfair? Your baby is finally asleep, but after being woken up for the umpteenth time during the night and despite feeling bone-weary tired, you just can't seem to fall asleep again. More than one-third of adults report symptoms of insomnia over the course of any given year, says the National Center for Sleep Disorders Research at the National Institutes of Health, and an unfortunate 10–15 percent of adults struggle with chronic insomnia.

You probably know the source of your sleep troubles (your newest family member, perhaps?), but additional contributors to insomnia include stress, anxiety, caffeine, or discomfort from a medical problem. Depression, work-shift issues, or travel may also be contributing factors. For some people, insomnia appears as trouble falling asleep, others have trouble staying asleep, and yet others may wake up too early —but it all comes down to not enough restorative sleep, which, in turn, leaves insomniacs feeling tired, irritable, and unfocused during the day.

Insomnia isn't just about tossing and turning during the night. People with insomnia may feel distressed during the day, fatigued, and develop memory problems. Studies indicate a strong link between insomnia and quality of life.[3] Insomniacs are more likely to have anxiety, depression, pain conditions, alcohol problems, and even heart disease.

Does getting enough high-quality sleep really matter? Absolutely! Well-rested people function better during the day, think more clearly, react more quickly, have better problem-solving skills, make better decisions, tend to be in a better mood, have a stronger immune system, have an easier time maintaining a healthy weight, and are just plain healthier. So whether one is born a "good sleeper" or turns to natural medicine to create a better sleep routine, the payoff is definitely worth it!

THE NATURAL SEARCH FOR SLEEP

Long before pharmaceutical sleeping pills came on the scene, herbs were the treatment of choice for restless nights. As a growing list of downsides from the use of sleeping pills becomes better known (such as interfering with natural sleep cycles and bestowing a "hangover" the next morning), herbal sleep aids again seem like the natural choice. Keep in mind that many of the natural sleep aids discussed in this chapter, especially the herbs, work well in concert and can readily be found in combination formulations.

5-HTP

Serotonin plays a big role in sleep, and 5-HTP helps the body make this chemical messenger. Studies have shown that taking 5-HTP helps resolve insomnia, bringing on better sleep quality and longer REM (rapid eye movement—the deepest form of sleep) sleep periods. The standard amount to take is 100–300 mg of 5-HTP before bedtime. Some people may feel a little nauseous when first taking 5-HTP, taking 50 mg the first few nights and building up to higher dosages may prevent this. There are some anecdotal reports of vivid dreams (and even nightmares) from taking large amounts of 5-HTP. Please note that people taking antidepressants (including SSRIs and MAO inhibitors) should not take 5-HTP.

Chamomile

Chamomile tea is a pleasant drink that has the added benefit of having a soothing, sedative effect. In addition to helping you unwind before bed, chamomile may also be used for anxiety and to soothe all manner of intestinal upset, such as indigestion and heartburn. Additional mildly sedating herbs include lemon balm, catnip, passion flower, and skull-cap. Passion flower should not be used during pregnancy, due to a risk of uterine contractions.

L-theanine

Green tea contains an amino acid, called L-theanine, that has a calming effect on the body and as an added bonus strengthens immunity. If feelings of anxiety interfere with sleep, taking 50–250 mg of L-theanine about an hour before your desired bedtime might help. L-theanine interacts with brain receptors associated with relaxation, inducing a relaxed state of mind.[4] L-theanine's general calming properties won't make a wired person suddenly fall asleep, but it may help quell feelings of anxiety so relaxation can ensue, which, in turn, promotes the ability to sleep.

L-tryptophan

The amino acid L-tryptophan is a precursor to the neurotransmitter serotonin, as well as melatonin. Three decades of research with L-tryptophan and sleep disorders show that 1–2 grams of this amino acid at bedtime shortens the time it takes to fall asleep and improves sleep quality, without interfering with cognitive performance.[5] As with 5-HTP, this supplement shouldn't be used by anyone taking antidepressants and should also be avoided by those with cirrhosis. L-tryptophan should not be taken during pregnancy because of concerns that this supplement could affect the breathing of a fetus or while nursing (due to a lack of safety data). This supplement was unavailable for several years, but is now back on the market.

Melatonin

The hormone melatonin plays an important role in regulating the body's clock, and it is secreted for several hours each night. As the sun sets, the pineal gland, located in the deepest recesses of the brain, begins to secrete the hormone melatonin. Melatonin levels remain high for the following eight to ten hours. But when sunlight hits the retinas—even through the eyelids—melatonin production is suppressed. The rise and fall of this amazing hormone figures prominently in the body's so-called circadian rhythm, which regulates our sleep/wake cycle.

People with insomnia tend to have lower levels of melatonin, as do shift workers and frequent flyers. Taking supplemental melatonin (particularly in the time-release form) an hour or so before desired bedtime may help all those groups get back into a better sleep schedule. Sleep experts generally recommended 3–5 mg of melatonin. Even as little as 0.5 mg helps convince the body that it's time to hit the hay. There are some reports of morning drowsiness with melatonin use. Side effects with melatonin are infrequent, although people with epilepsy should not take this hormone because of concerns that melatonin may increase seizures and those taking warfarin should not use melatonin because it could increase the risk of bleeding. Due to a lack of safety data, do not take melatonin while you're pregnant or nursing.

Valerian

Valerian is the standout among herbal sleep aids; it's been bestowing sweet dreams for herbally inclined insomniacs for more than a thousand years. Valerian, in the amount of 500 mg of an herbal extract taken before bed, eases stress and has a scientifically documented sedative effect, yet it's nonaddictive, and there is no morning hangover from using it. One study found that taking valerian extract reduced the time it took to fall to sleep on a par with that found when using prescription sedatives. According to research, a combination of valerian and hops helps "bad sleepers" finally nod off.[6] The forty-two people in this double-blind, placebo-controlled study did not have any sleep-affecting diseases (such as sleep apnea), but they all had a history of tossing and turning. On the nights these insomniacs took a valerian-hops combination, they not only slept longer, but they also experienced deeper sleep, compared to those on placebo.

IS SNORING THE CULPRIT?

I have a confession: I am a very noisy snorer during the final months of pregnancy or when I'm sick with a cold. But, luckily, not so much at other times. My husband battles with insomnia on a regular basis, and I don't think my snoring does him any favors. This scenario is repeated in bedrooms all around the world. The insomnia of one person is directly related to the snoring of the other. In fact, bed partners of people who snore lose up to an hour of sleep each night.

For the millions of Americans who snore (plus the millions more sleeping next to these noisy nappers), snoring is a relatively minor health problem that may negatively affect a surprisingly large part of waking life. The loss of deep, restorative sleep for both the snorer and the "snoree" may lead to daytime sleepiness, difficulty concentrating, crankiness, and an increased risk of car accidents.

Better sleep all around can be achieved by treating the partner's snoring. First, treat or rule out health conditions that may be causing your snoring, such as sleep apnea, hypothyroidism, allergies, or a deviated septum. However, for most snorers, there is no known cause for sawing logs. It is simply caused by the sound of inhaled air vibrating against floppy tissues of the throat, much like the rattling of windows in an old house on a windy night. The vibrations tend to be localized along either the uvula (the little piece of pink tissue dangling in the back of the throat) or the soft palate.

What Makes People Snore?

Why does snoring only occur at night, even though air is inhaled around the clock? Because during waking hours, the brain keeps the throat muscles adequately tightened to prevent the floppy, noisy vibrations. The brain lets down its guard during the relaxation of sleep, and snoring noises are heard.

The older you get, the more likely you are to be a snorer. By the age of fifty, half of men and a quarter of women snore. Packing on a few extra pounds adds to the problem, since there are more tissues around the neck area available to vibrate. The snoring-obesity connection is so clear-cut that losing weight is considered one of the best ways to turn down the racket.

Anything that makes the throat muscles relax more than usual or causes the throat tissues to swell or narrow makes for an extra-noisy night of snoring. What's on such a list of snore-aggravators? Alcohol, tranquilizers, cigarettes, sleep deprivation, the common cold, hay fever, and pregnancy are the biggies here.

How you sleep may even contribute to whether or not you snore. Lying flat on your back allows the tongue to fall backward and block part of the airway, thus bringing on snoring. Sleeping on your side might quiet things down.

UNDERSTANDING CHRONIC FATIGUE SYNDROME

While everyone feels tired sometimes (especially new parents!), chronic fatigue syndrome (CFS) is this "average" level of weariness taken to radical lengths—to the point where fatigue hampers the completion of basic daily activities. CFS is not a single entity; rather, it's a collection of symptoms that range from physical symptoms of muscle fatigue, exhaustion, joint aches, fever, night sweats, and sore throat to mental and emotional symptoms of depression, insomnia, and poor concentration. These symptoms persist for months or even years and interfere with day-to-day life.

CFS has long been a mystery condition. The underlying cause of CFS remains unknown; furthermore, it was only within the last couple of decades that it was even acknowledged as a legitimate health condition by the Centers for Disease Control and Prevention. Regardless of its recent acceptance into the fold of official diseases, it seems to have existed in the past in many different incarnations, from "effort syndrome" in World War I veterans and "the vapors" in nineteenth-century women to, more recently, hypoglycemia and chronic mononucleosis.

More than 2 million Americans—most frequently young, white, professional women—are estimated to suffer from CFS. For many people, a viral infection, such as the Epstein-Barr virus, precedes the onset of CFS. According to the official diagnostic criteria, CFS is present when a person experiences persistent fatigue for at least six months as well as four or more of the following symptoms:

- Impaired short-term memory or concentration severe enough to interfere with usual activities

- Sore throat

- Swollen lymph nodes

- Muscle and/or joint pain without joint swelling or redness

- Headaches

- Unrefreshing sleep

- Postexertion weariness lasting more than 24 hours

Since many other health conditions, such as Lyme disease, cancer, bacterial infection, autoimmune disease, or HIV (human immunodeficiency virus), have symptoms similar to CFS, they should be ruled out before CFS is diagnosed.

Natural Ways to Alleviate CFS

General improvements in lifestyle, as well as stress management techniques, may combat some of the symptoms of CFS. On the other hand, poor health habits, such as smoking, an unbalanced diet, excessive alcohol consumption, and lack of exercise, may aggravate CFS symptoms. Although exercise is probably the last thing fatigued people feel like doing, research shows that moderate exercise may be a valuable part of a CFS treatment protocol; for many CFS sufferers, regular exercise prevents the fatigue from worsening. However, exercise seems to make the condition worse in some individuals.

Maintaining a healthy immune system is another valuable tool for preventing and treating CFS. A broad range of nutrients are important to a vigilant, well-functioning immune system. In particular, the antioxidants (vitamins A, C, E, and the carotenoids) help maintain and repair the immune system. The B vitamins, vitamin D, zinc, copper, selenium, the bioflavonoids, and essential fatty acids also figure prominently in proper immune function.

The mineral magnesium plays an integral role in energy production, since it is needed to convert carbohydrates, protein, and fats into energy. People suffering from CFS tend to have low blood levels of magnesium. Furthermore, CFS patients taking magnesium supplements report greater energy levels, improved emotional state, and less pain than those taking a placebo.

CFS patients report an improvement in symptoms when supplementing with essential fatty acids daily for three months (a mix of EPA and DHA from fish oil, as well as gamma-linolenic acid).[7]

L-carnitine, an amino acid, is needed for the production of energy in the mitochondria of cells. Some researchers suspect that individuals with CFS may have mitochondria that do not function properly. Accordingly, deficiencies of L-carnitine have been reported in some people with CFS. Even more suggestive is a study that found that 3 grams of L-carnitine daily may alleviate some of the symptoms of CFS.[8]

Coenzyme Q_{10} may also be important for those with CFS. Coenzyme Q_{10} is concentrated in the mitochondria, where it is crucial for energy production. Although there have not been any studies with coenzyme Q_{10} and CFS sufferers, several researchers suspect that there may be a link.

RESTLESS LEG SYNDROME

You finally sit down to relax with a book or lie down for the night, and that's when it starts. Creepy, crawly sensations in your legs that demand your attention, triggering an uncontrollable urge to move your legs. Up to 12 million Americans have restless leg syndrome (RLS), which causes these unpleasant sensations in the legs. Sounds mild, but for many people with RLS, it interferes with sleep, work, relationships, and quality of life.

RLS is fairly uncommon before pregnancy, but by the third trimester about one-quarter of women complain of it. It seems that women with lower blood levels of folic acid are most likely to end up with RLS.[9] In addition, RLS tends to run in families, and people with genetically related RLS appear to have inherited an unusually high requirement for folic acid. In one report, forty-five people were identified to be from families with folic acid–responsive RLS. The amount of folic acid required to relieve their symptoms was extremely large, ranging from 5,000 to 30,000 mcg per day. Such amounts should *only* be taken under the supervision of a health care professional.

People with low iron levels may be prone to developing RLS, and increasing iron intake may result in fewer symptoms. But iron won't help RLS unless you are deficient in iron (and you shouldn't take extra iron unless you are deficient). If you suspect that your RLS is related to a low iron level, consider having your iron tested.

Keep in mind, however, that the most commonly used iron tests (both the hemoglobin and hematocrit tests) are best for showing the late stages of iron deficiency, called anemia. Mild or moderate deficiencies, which are more common, are best found with other tests, such as the serum ferritin, serum iron, transferrin saturation, or transferrin receptor test, which you can ask your doctor to order.

In a preliminary trial, people with RLS who suffered from insomnia had a significant improvement in sleep efficiency after supplementing with magnesium (about 300 mg each evening for four to six weeks).

Caffeine and alcohol may aggravate or trigger symptoms in those who are predisposed to develop RLS. Some studies have shown that a reduction or complete elimination of such substances may relieve symptoms.

CHAPTER 9

Stress and Sanity

Staying focused, joyful, and calm may be the biggest challenge for new parents. Although you love your new child beyond measure, there's also a reason for the saying "It's a good thing you're cute." You'll probably be thinking or saying that a lot during the challenging times of new motherhood, when faced with a crying, fussy baby or a crabby, obstinate toddler. This chapter will give you some tools to help navigate the mental waters of new parenthood: the depression, anxiety, stress, and mental dullness that all too often appear when a baby joins a family.

IS THERE NO ESCAPING THE BABY BLUES?

It's not a matter of *if* you're going to get the baby blues, but *when* and *how bad.* Up to 80 percent of new moms experience the baby blues as at least a mildly lousy mood in the few days after giving birth, and oftentimes it is far worse. Baby blues trigger feelings of irritability, sadness, anxiety, confusion, being overwhelmed, and being incompetent, as well as crying episodes, mood swings, and changes in appetite and sleep patterns. Baby blues generally peak in the first week or so after delivery and go away after a few days or weeks. It is extremely common and— once again—linked to the hormone roller coaster of the postpartum period. Of course, the heady new responsibilities of taking care of a new person also contribute to the intensity of the situation.

Mood changes that are severe (called postpartum depression, or PPD for short) only occur in about 10 percent of women. If you have a history of severe PMS, thyroid problems, or depression, you're more likely to be one of the unlucky moms hit with postpartum depression. It may be challenging to determine the difference between baby blues and outright depression. There are a few key differences. First, the timing may be a clue. The blues develop soon after birth and go away in a few days (or they might stretch on for weeks). Second, baby blues are less severe than outright depression. Although you experience sadness and negative emotions, it is still possible for you to get through your day and keep up with all your responsibilities. With postpartum depression, your daily functioning is impaired.

Finally, consider your risk factors. Any woman is vulnerable to the baby blues, but if you have a personal or family history of depression, you should definitely take that into account. In terms of treatment, the baby blues go away on their own, but depression requires medical attention.

Well, you may be thinking, that's great that the baby blues will go away on their own, but can't I still get a little TLC during this trying time? Absolutely! First and foremost, try to get as much sleep as you can (yes, I know that is asking for the near-impossible). But the sad fact is that sleep deprivation will magnify your emotional upheaval. Nap when your baby naps and say yes if a friend or family member offers some help with your new baby. Sleep deprivation is a major risk factor in PPD.

In the midst of emotional upheaval with the baby blues, the following advice may be very tough to follow, but getting out and exercising is a great way to activate your happiness endorphins. Even a very slow, gentle exercise, such as tai chi, may help alleviate depression and lift your mood.[1] If you're still feeling "beat up" from the birth process, a slow walk around the block might be all you are up to, but even that may help.

Remember, the baby blues are generally a temporary occurrence;

Symptoms of Postpartum Depression

- Apathy
- Lethargy
- Persistent feelings of sadness
- Insomnia
- Loss of appetite
- Feeling disconnected from your newborn
- Memory loss
- Severe anxiety
- Bouts of crying
- Withdrawal from family and friends
- Thoughts of harming yourself or your baby

The general rule is if a new mom has one or more of the above symptoms for more than two weeks, then postpartum depression is considered as a diagnosis.

your crazy mood will pass and you will feel emotionally settled again in the near future. However, if your baby blues continue for more than a few weeks, call your doctor. Other organizations that can help include Postpartum Support International (postpartum.net) and Postpartum Education for Parents (sbpep.org).

WHY WOMEN OUTNUMBER MEN
WHEN IT COMES TO MOOD PROBLEMS

Women outnumber men two to one in terms of depression, but why? Not only are more women depressed than men, but the depressions women experience last longer and are less likely to resolve themselves without treatment. Statistics show that one in every seven women will suffer from at least one episode of depression in her life. Many experts believe that hormones account for a large part of the gender difference in depression. Hormonal roller coasters during the menstrual cycle, during and after pregnancy, and during the use of oral contraceptives may all impact a woman's mood.

Other factors that may account for the disproportionately higher incidence of depression in women include the need to juggle work and family demands, the stress of single parenthood, and financial inequality.

HOW OMEGA-3 HELPS

The omega-3 fatty acids found in fish oil may play a role in mood during the first years of new motherhood.[2] It is known that women with lower tissue levels of the omega-3 fatty acid called DHA are more likely to develop postpartum depression. To make matters worse, the physical demands of pregnancy and breast-feeding drain a woman's reserve of DHA from the brain, leaving her vulnerable to mood-related health problems. By contrast, women with greater fish consumption are shown in studies to be less likely to have PPD. Eating fish twice a week or supplementing with omega-3 through pregnancy and while lactating makes sense as a way to lessen the risk of depression.

EXERCISE LIFTS MOOD

In general, people who are depressed benefit from exercise, and the same is true for new moms facing the baby blues. Women who are more active in the weeks and months after giving birth report more satisfaction with motherhood overall. Even a single session of exercise has been shown to lead to more positive feelings (including positive mood, better energy level, happiness, and a feeling of being refreshed) and a decrease in tension, anxiety, and confusion. Aerobic exercise, such as walking, running, cycling, or swimming, provides a stronger mood lift than anaerobic activities, such as weight lifting.

When new mothers participated in a study comparing an exercise program with parenting education to education alone, the women who engaged in exercise showed significant benefits in terms of depression symptoms and feelings of well-being. The number of women identified as "at risk" for postpartum depression was reduced by 50 percent in the exercise group by the end of the study.[3]

SPECIAL ADVICE FOR THOSE TAKING ANTIDEPRESSANTS

Some of the most popular antidepressants today—including fluoxetine (Prozac)—are what is known as selective serotonin reuptake inhibitor (SSRI) drugs. SSRI drugs work by keeping more serotonin (a brain chemical that plays an important role in mood) in the brain.

Not everyone feels better when taking fluoxetine for depression, and experts have discovered that people who have low levels of folic acid in their bodies are more likely to be in this nonresponder group.[4] Simply taking folic acid (200–500 mcg per day) with the antidepressant leads to significantly greater response to the drug. This amount of folic acid is the amount present in most daily multivitamins. Experts believe that folic acid supplements improve the antidepressant action of other antidepressant drugs as well.

ST. JOHN'S WORT FOR DEPRESSION

St. John's wort's sunny appearance, due to its golden-yellow, perky flowers, brightens up a room, but the extract from this herb is what's really effective in battling the blues. Studies document that this herb is as effective as prescription drugs for mild to moderate depression, with the added benefit of not causing the sleep and sexual side effects of prescription antidepressants.[5]

Okay, St. John's wort does have to own up to a few things. Since St. John's wort makes the skin more sensitive to light, fair-skinned individuals taking this herb should avoid strong sunlight and tanning beds (but, seriously, you should avoid tanning beds regardless of taking this herb!). Also, St. John's wort may negatively interact with compounds in certain foods like red wine, aged cheese, yeast, and pickled herring, which is why these foods should be avoided. And remember, St. John's wort should not be taken in combination with antidepressant medications.

Other Natural Depression Treatments

The B vitamins may be just the ticket for some downhearted women, especially for those taking the Pill. Birth control pills may deplete the body's stores of vitamin B_6, which, in turn, affects the production of mood-altering brain chemicals. Women who develop depression while taking birth control pills sometimes perk up after supplementing with vitamin B_6 (start out with 20 mg twice daily). Extra vitamin B_6 may also be the answer for women whose depression is linked to PMS.

But you don't have to be on the Pill or plagued with PMS to come up short when it comes to vitamin B_6. Harvard scientists found that, in a group of depressed but otherwise healthy young adults, more than one in four were deficient in vitamin B_6, as well as vitamins B_{12} and riboflavin.[6] Other researchers concur that low levels of vitamin B_{12} may interfere with mood, while supplements of this vitamin may brighten spirits.

Another B vitamin, folic acid, is also implicated in depression, since as many as one-third of depressed individuals have marginal or deficient folic acid levels, and moods improve with folic acid supplements. When the blood levels of folic acid are compared in those in healthy people of all ages, those with the highest levels report the best moods, while those with lower levels are more likely to be depressed.

With the B vitamins, if you're missing one, chances are good that other B vitamins are also on the low side. Which is why it makes sense to take a B-complex supplement to cover all the bases if you're feeling down in the dumps.

Minerals may also account for mood ups and downs. For example, when researchers track the moods of people who consume a low-selenium or high-selenium diet, they find that moods match the selenium level of the diet.[7] Iron deficiency may be linked to depression, as well.

ANXIOUS MOTHERHOOD

You pace around the room with your thoughts racing, drum your fingers on the table, or perhaps sit quietly while the pressure seems to be building to unbearable levels around you. Whatever the underlying trigger, this feeling of anxiety is one that everyone has experienced at one time or another. Being a new mother tends to send anxiety into overdrive—you're responsible for an entire life, after all. Lisa, the mother of a five-month-old and a three-year-old, definitely notices an uptick of anxiety in her life since becoming a parent. "I can't go to sleep myself until I have checked that all the doors in the house are locked, which may be normal, but I also can't go to sleep until I've checked that both kids are breathing," she explains. Turns out, that's pretty normal, too.

Although jangled nerves may be unsettling, anxiety in some situations does heighten the body's ability to focus, concentrate, and complete the task at hand. However, for many people—some experts suggest up to 8 percent of the population—anxiety and nervousness become overriding factors in their lives and impair their ability to function optimally at work and socially. These people experience extended periods of worry and intense fear, which is out of proportion to the situation they are facing. In some cases there is no basis for worry, but feelings of anxiety are present nonetheless.

While most Americans suffering from anxiety disorders are plied with tranquilizers or other addictive (and side-effect-causing) drugs, there are natural anti-anxiety alternatives.

Playing Mind Games

Visualizing success is a great way to keep life lighthearted. Worrying that is letting your mind focus on what could go wrong in your life, instead of focusing on what might go right, unconsciously sets you up for failure and cranks up your anxiety level. Your body reacts to the mental imagery of an unloving day-care provider, losing your job, a conflict with your mate, or any other imagined problem, as if the situation were actually happening; stress hormones are pumped out of your adrenals, your heart rate increases, and your muscles tense. By directing your mental imagery toward visualizing success, your body relaxes, you feel better, and your unconscious mind works to reach these positive goals.

Stress management techniques that calm the inner environment go a long way toward helping you deal with the hectic outside world. Meditation is one such coping mechanism that has both a long history and modern confirmation of its effectiveness. By working to quiet the mind and body, meditation reduces the sometimes overwhelming stimulation that drives feelings of anxiety and stress. Meditation comes in many varieties, but they all boil down to two basic techniques: inducing a quiet body and a quiet mind. An easy approach to meditation is to sit or lie down in a dark room and then focus on a word or phrase as you breathe in and out deeply and evenly for about twenty minutes.

A New Way to Un-Panic

Panic attacks are a type of anxiety disorder that may come on suddenly and without warning, leaving a person panting, with a pounding heart, and feeling very anxious. The supplement inositol (a member of the B-complex family of vitamins) has been found to quell the frequency and severity of panic attacks, as well as episodes of agoraphobia (fear of open or public places). People with obsessive-compulsive disorder have also shown improvement with inositol supplements. Most studies with inositol have called for subjects to take 12–18 grams per day, an amount that has not been associated with any adverse effects, although this supplement should not be used during pregnancy, as it may induce contractions.

Herbs and Supplements for Anxiety

The B-complex vitamins play a role in how well—or how poorly—your body responds to the pressures of modern living. For starters, most of the B vitamins are involved in a well-functioning nervous system. B-complex supplements may help ensure that the nervous system is up to the challenge of life's ups and downs. Since nutritional surveys suggest that many American diets fall short of several of the B vitamins, a balanced B-complex supplement may be both a form of general nutritional insurance and a way to boost the body's resistance to the effects of stress.

Of the B-complex vitamins, vitamin B_3 in the form called niacinamide may be particularly beneficial, since it seems to have a similar effect in the brain as certain conventional anti-anxiety drugs (such as Valium). Supplements providing 500 mg of niacinamide several times daily may ease anxiety and stress.

Sitting down to enjoy a cup of tea is certainly a soothing ritual, but if it's green tea in your cup, there's even more reason to feel calm. Green tea contains a compound called L-theanine that acts as a natural stress reliever, in addition to counteracting the stimulant effects of caffeine and keeping blood pressure in check. Certain neurotransmitters (namely, serotonin and dopamine) are altered after L-theanine enters the body, and it's these changes in the brain that trigger relaxation without a loss of clear thinking. In other words, L-theanine relaxes the mind without causing any drowsiness. The ability to focus on taxing mental exercises increases with L-theanine, even while wound-up feelings unwind themselves.

Many herbs have a calming effect. For example, valerian eases stress and has a mild sedating influence on the central nervous system; chamomile also has a soothing effect. Oat straw, hops, and passion flower have been employed traditionally by herbalists to help calm anxious or burned-out people. Passion flower should not be used during pregnancy, due to a risk of uterine contractions. St. John's wort may also play a role in managing stress.

STRESS DURING BABY'S FIRST YEAR

Even for people who haven't just become new parents, up to 90 percent of doctor visits are connected to stress in some way. Stress is a factor in an astounding number of health conditions: from headaches and depression to stomach upset, heart disease, and compromised immune function. Stress even affects how long you'll live, since chronic stress lowers longevity. Not all stress is bad, of course; some stress serves as a motivator to complete important tasks (such as jumping out of bed at 2 a.m. to comfort a crying baby). However, excessive stress results in damaging wear and tear on body, mind, and soul.

To add yet another strain to marriages after a baby joins the family, stress is the nemesis of a healthy sex drive. The fight-or-flight response of adrenaline cuts blood flow to "nonessential" body parts, and, in this case, that includes the genitals. Being wound up and stressed out is just not compatible with great sex.

MEDITATION AND EXERCISE

Stress management techniques that calm the inner environment can go a long way toward helping you deal with the hectic outside world. As with anxiety, meditation eases stress. After twenty minutes of meditation, you may find that you have a whole new perspective on the things stressing you out.

And don't forget about one other stress reliever: sex. Sex is actually a very effective way to lower your stress level; you just have to find the time to partake in this pleasure.

Exercise is a great outlet for tension that builds up during times of anxiety and stress. Sudden, short-term bouts of anxiety are more responsive to exercise than are chronic feelings of anxiety. Physical activity is such a great way to manage tension that researchers have even found that regular exercise provides as much benefit as meditation and other relaxation techniques when it comes to alleviating anxiety.

SUPPLEMENTS AND HERBS TO DE-STRESS

Stress and anxiety take their toll on mineral stores in the body. Type A people—the archetype of highly stressed individuals—have been found to have higher levels of stress hormones in their blood, yet lower levels of magnesium when compared to their more laid-back counterparts. As if that weren't enough, these stress hormones cause body cells to lose magnesium. And as the body's stores of magnesium are drained, the stress response is activated—leading to a stress spiral. All of this, of course, does not promote a sense of relaxation.

Most people do not consume recommended intake levels of magnesium in their diets. Researchers have found that 200 mg of magnesium daily (combined with 50 mg of vitamin B_6) is very helpful in relieving PMS-related anxiety in women.[8] Wound up, anxious folks tend to have lower levels of the essential fatty acid omega-3. Meanwhile, supplementing with omega-3—which can be found in fish oil—dials down the body's stress pathways.[9]

Supplementing with omega-3 helps adults cope with the normal pressures in life and even keeps stress in check during high-stress periods (researchers demonstrated this benefit by giving university students fish oil supplements during their final exams).[10] The American Psychiatric Association (APA) recognizes the important connection between omega-3s and mental health by recommending that all adults get at least two servings of fish a week. For those with mood and anxiety issues, consuming enough omega-3s is even more crucial, which is why the APA recommends at least 1,000 mg of EPA and DHA daily in this group.

Adaptogenic herbs—those that serve as a general tonic and promote overall wellness and vitality—come to the rescue in times of stress by enabling the body to deal with stressful situations in a more effective manner. Asian ginseng represents the best-known of the adaptogenic herbs, but there are others that deserve consideration in terms of their stress management properties, including ashwagandha and rhodiola. Asian ginseng inhibits the production of stress hormones, ashwagandha provides a sense of calm on par with prescription anti-anxiety drugs, and rhodiola has been shown to fortify the body against both physical and mental stressors.[11] Ginseng shouldn't be used during pregnancy since there is research questioning this herb's safety in terms of birth defects. It should also be avoided by nursing women because there is no safety data associated with this herb during lactation.

Vitamin C is one of the first nutrients to be affected by physical or emotional stress. To make matters worse, depleted levels of vitamin C may interfere with proper immune function, leaving the body vulnerable to infection—which then acts as yet another stressor on the body. Adding insult to injury, the stress glands (such as the adrenals and the pituitary) are among the repositories of vitamin C, so stress may drain the body's stores of vitamin C.

MOMMY BRAIN

Some people call it "mommy brain," but however you refer to it, it's no fun feeling as though your IQ plummeted once you had a baby. Much of your foggy thinking is connected to lost sleep and extra responsibilities. Stress is another major brain drainer. Individuals under stress often develop short-term memory problems, difficulty concentrating, and attention deficits.

A few weeks after new mom Jessica went back to work after maternity leave, she experienced quite the "mommy meltdown moment." She laughs, remembering this particular day (after several low-sleep nights): "I left my briefcase at the day-care center, brought the diaper bag into my office, picked up the telephone, and dialed my calculator." You won't feel this spacey forever. In the meantime, however, if you want to regain your mental prowess, there are natural products that may help.

Acetyl-L-carnitine

Acetyl-L-carnitine is a beneficial supplement for clearer thinking. Acetyl-L-carnitine contributes the acetyl molecule, which is required in the manufacture of the brain transmitter acetylcholine. Too little acetylcholine, which is necessary in the formation of memories, is a main factor in declining memory function. Acetyl-L-carnitine contributes to healthy brain function in another way: it eliminates fatty acids from the brain, which would become toxic if they were allowed to accumulate. You can try 500 mg of acetyl-L-carnitine, three times per day.

Citicoline

Citicoline supplements have been shown to increase energy in the part of the brain responsible for focus and concentration. Recently, Harvard researchers supplemented healthy men and women with 500–2,000 mg of citicoline daily for six weeks. Results indicated higher energy reserves in the all-important frontal lobe of the brain, the area of mental focus.[12]

Curcumin

Curcumin, extracted from the herb tumeric, improves memory and learning ability in animals. Curcumin also benefits the aging brain by blocking certain changes and cell death that would otherwise negatively impact cognition and memory. You might notice sharper thinking when taking 500–1,000 mg per day. High amounts of curcumin during pregnancy could theoretically trigger contractions, so it should not be used in pregnancy.

Ginkgo

Ginkgo, taken alone and in various combinations with other supplements, has a large body of research showing beneficial effects on cognition. It is used in the amount of 120–240 mg per day. However, do not take ginkgo if you're pregnant or nursing as its safety during those times has not been established.

Huperzine

Numerous herbs—backed by both a long tradition of use and scientific research—have the potential to enhance thinking powers. For example, the supplement huperzine comes from a type of Chinese moss and is used for age-related cognitive decline. It works by preventing the breakdown of the neurotransmitter acetylcholine. Huperzine has been used in China as a folk remedy to enhance mental abilities, and modern research indicates positive effects for patients with dementia. It can be safely used in the amount of 200–600 mcg per day.

Iron

Quick—name three words to describe anemia. Do the words *pale, tired, and weak* come to mind? New research suggests that if you had trouble completing this mental exercise, that in itself may be a symptom of the early stages of anemia.

Iron deficiency may impair thinking processes, while iron supplements (in iron-deficient individuals) may boost memory and the ability to learn. Iron deficiency is most prevalent in teenage girls and women in their childbearing years.

Iron deficiency, even before anemia develops, may cause many health problems, such as decreased endurance, lowered work capacity, and depressed immune function. Supplements of iron may alleviate many of these physical complications of iron deficiency, as well as the cognitive symptoms, such as impaired learning ability and memory. The amount of iron in a multivitamin/mineral (which is generally 18 mg) is fine to take, but more than that should only be taken if your doctor diagnoses iron deficiency.

Omega-3 Fatty Acids

The human brain is composed of a significant amount of fat, which it needs to run properly. Supplementing with the right fats helps make sure everything keeps humming along. Omega-3 fatty acids contribute a lot to the brain, such as providing nutrients critical for the structure and function of brain cells. Research indicates that regular consumption of the omega-3 fatty acids EPA and DHA results in improved cognition and better memory. Try a supplement supplying at least 500 mg (of EPA and DHA) per day.

Phosphatidylserine

A specialized type of fat called phosphatidylserine (PS) is found in brain cell membranes, where it facilitates communication between brain cells to aid memory and clear thinking. Clinical research has focused on PS for several decades, particularly in connection to cognitive function. According to studies with PS, this supplement (used in the amount of 300 mg per day) not only safeguards brain function in older adults, it may counteract some age-related cognitive decline as well.[13] PS, combined with the herb ginkgo, improves memory performance in people, especially when they are given tasks that must be completed quickly.[14]

Pycnogenol

Supplements of pycnogenol (pine bark extract) contain antioxidant bioflavonoids that positively affect cognitive measures. A study of 101 elderly participants found that a daily supplement of 150 mg of pycnogenol (compared to a placebo) for three months enhanced subjects' ability to perform cognitive tasks and increased attention, working memory, and episodic memory.[15]

Rhodiola

Rhodiola, an herb that sometimes goes by the name golden root, has been used traditionally in Russia for energy. Research (both in Russia and the United States) indicates that rhodiola improves cognitive function, particularly during times of stress. Try 200–600 mg of a standardized extract before each meal.

Vinpocetine

Vinpocetine is an extract from the periwinkle plant. In addition to being an antioxidant, vinpocetine relaxes blood vessels and thins the blood, thereby increasing blood flow to the brain. During supplementation with vinpocetine, in the amount of 10–30 mg per day, the brain becomes enriched with oxygen. Scientific trials of adults with mild cognitive impairment supplementing with vinpocetine show improvements in memory, learning, and overall cognitive performance.[16]

Vitamin B_{12}

Vitamin B_{12} is critical for cognitive function, and deficiencies of this vitamin are too often underdiagnosed. Supplementing with 1,000 mcg of vitamin B_{12} may lead to improvements in cognitive function.

THE RETURN OF YOUR PERIOD . . . AND PMS

For women who don't breast-feed, expect your period to return six to eight weeks after giving birth. For breast-feeding moms, you'll get a longer reprieve of numerous months and perhaps even for as long as you're nursing. But remember, even if your period hasn't returned, you can still get pregnant! Ovulation occurs a few weeks before your period returns, so always use birth control if you aren't ready for another baby yet. When your period does finally return, it's normal for it to be irregular for the first few cycles.

And now that your period is returning, get ready for premenstrual syndrome (PMS). Three out of four women experience PMS during their reproductive years, especially during their twenties and thirties. More than 150 different symptoms have been documented in women suffering from PMS, but most PMS sufferers note that their symptoms of pain, mood changes, weight gain, swelling, breast tenderness, and cravings develop one to fourteen days prior to menstruation.

Natural Ways to Ease PMS

An imbalance in the female hormone estrogen, as well as progesterone, might be a contributing factor in PMS. Exercise is an excellent first-line natural remedy to reestablish balance when estrogen levels are out of whack. Regular exercise lowers circulating levels of estrogen, not to mention all the other health perks that come from hitting the gym.[17] After the ovaries, the top producer of estrogen is fat cells. Women with greater stores of body fat have higher estrogen levels, so it follows that exercising away fat stores also gets rid of extra estrogen. Not surprisingly, how much fat is in your diet also influences fat stores, and thus estrogen levels. And don't forget about fiber, since a high-fiber diet enhances estrogen excretion and can thereby improve hormonal balance and alleviate PMS symptoms. Most women don't even get half the 28 grams of fiber they should eat every day. Among other dietary changes, some women find PMS relief from avoiding any sources of caffeine.

The roles of the hormones estrogen and progesterone are intertwined, with each serving as a check and balance for the other. The herb vitex (also known as chasteberry) is a go-to herb for PMS, because it naturally ups production of progesterone, thereby balancing out estrogen. Take note, however, that vitex is not quick-acting. It may take several months to ease your symptoms, and it should be discontinued if you become pregnant, since there is a slight concern that this herb (by encouraging menstruation) could interfere with pregnancy.

Depending on the particular symptoms you experience, various nutrients may be of help. Among the most effective supplements for PMS are vitamin B_6, evening primrose oil, vitamin E, and magnesium.

RETURNING TO WORK

A mama's got to do what a mama's got to do. If you are going the road alone or your income is part of the team effort it takes to pay the bills, then you might just have to jump back into work life after your six weeks of maternity leave. Remind yourself (as often as needed) that the emotional bond between mother and child survives hours apart.

Cut yourself some slack. Even without adding the ball of "work," you are juggling a lot of new responsibilities with a new baby. It's natural and normal to have intense emotions at times, including sadness, guilt, or even relief. Working or not, guilt is the emotion that seems to connect all mothers.

If you are fortunate enough to have a bit of flexibility at work (and in your budget), the following ideas may make your transition back to the workforce a bit easier for you and your baby:

- Can you switch to part time or perhaps change to a job-share, in which you and a coworker each work the same job part time?

- Make your reentry a bit smoother by working just a few days a week for your first month back.

- Set up some flex time. For example, starting work earlier in the day so you get done in the afternoon could give you more time with your baby during his or her waking hours.

- Eat at your desk. If you can cut out your lunch hour, you could head home that much earlier at the end of the day. Not possible with your work? Then squeeze in all the errands and chores that you can during your lunch hour to give you more downtime at home. For example, working mom Kelley does her grocery shopping during lunch (stashing the cold items in the office fridge) so that her evenings are less hectic at home with her child.

- Can you work from home a few days a week?

- Can you afford to take a longer leave from work—will your boss allow it? You might want to remind your company that it costs between 75 percent and 200 percent of your salary to replace you.

- Find a day-care center close to your workplace so you can visit your baby during the day.

CHAPTER 10

After-Baby Health Concerns

I t's tough enough to keep slogging through your days when your nights are kept busy with baby needs, but adding new health problems for yourself into the mix can make you feel utterly overwhelmed. From backaches and headaches to hemorrhoids, bladder troubles, and yeast infections, there's a lot of physical discomfort that new moms may face. Find some relief with the natural remedies discussed in this chapter.

ASTHMA

In the past decade or so, asthma has become more prevalent than ever before and now afflicts more than 17 million people in the United States—8 percent of the population. With asthma, the airways become swollen and inflamed, resulting in wheezing, coughing, chest tightness, and difficulty breathing. Common asthma triggers include viral illness; cigarette smoke; air pollution; allergens, such as dust mites, pollen, mold, or animal dander; and even such things as exercise, stress, cold temperatures, and the use of aspirin.

Natural medicine offers some alternatives that may help keep asthma at bay and reduce reliance on conventional (and side effect–ridden) asthma medications. Low levels of vitamin D are considered a culprit in asthma. Vitamin D improves lung function, as well as supporting a strong immune system. For adults, 1,000–2,000 IU daily of vitamin D is a helpful amount.

People with asthma can sometimes reduce their reliance on inhaled corticosteroids when supplementing with 1,000 mg of vitamin C daily.[1] Vitamin C supports the body's own production of corticosteroids in the adrenal glands. By taking lower doses of corticosteroids (and still keeping asthma under control), you lessen the risks of side effects, such as cataracts, bone loss, and immune system suppression. *Note:* Do not abruptly discontinue steroid medications; work with a doctor to safely adjust your dosage downward.

Boswellia, also known as frankincense, is a tree found in India, North Africa, and the Middle East. A gummy resin taken from the tree bark blocks the synthesis of proinflammatory compounds that have a role in an asthma attack's constriction of the bronchials, which reduces airflow in and out of the lungs. In short, boswellia gets to source of the problem to prevent the cause of an acute asthma attack. Consider taking 300 mg, three times a day.

A European herb called butterbur has been lauded for easing asthma symptoms ever since the seventeenth century. Modern research indicates that butterbur soothes airway spasms; one study found that more than 40 percent of butterbur users were able to take less asthma medication, while keeping asthma symptoms under control.[2,3] To try butterbur, take 50–100 mg twice a day with meals. Make sure to select a product that contains no pyrrolizidine alkaloids (compounds that can cause liver damage).

BACK HEALTH

About 80 percent of Americans will suffer from back pain at some time in their lives, and it's easy to see why new parents are at extra risk, with all the bending, lifting, and holding of babies. In fact, low-back pain is the second most common reason for visits to a primary care physician, outnumbered only by the common cold. You don't have to wait until you become another back pain statistic; there are many ways to keep your back healthy and pain-free.

A sedentary lifestyle contributes to the development of back pain, while keeping active helps maintain a healthy back. Walking is an excellent exercise for prevention (and sometimes treatment) of low back pain because it helps to tone the muscles that keep us upright, thus helping to maintain proper posture.

While everyone knows how to walk, you might not be doing it in the best form. You should give yourself a quick assessment to check if you are walking with erect posture, your head level and your feet shoulder-width apart. If seen from the side, your ear should be aligned with your shoulders and hips. If these body structures do not align, there may be some abnormalities in the curves of the spine. Aim for ten thousand steps—this is about thirty minutes of walking—every day.

The position you sleep in may affect how you feel when you get up in the morning (assuming, of course, that your baby is letting you sleep!). A side-lying sleeping posture is best for most people. Try placing a pillow under your head just high enough to keep the head level and firm enough that it is the same height when you turn over. And try a second pillow for between your knees. This keeps the body straight and the spine aligned while you sleep. In terms of the bed's mattress, while mattress preference is a personal matter, most people with back pain find that a medium-hard mattress gives the best support and minimizes any curve in the spine.

With the wrong shoes, your back could pay the consequences. High heels, especially when worn over a period of years, can cause significant changes in the structure of the foot and the arches, and this elevation of the heel changes the curves of the lumbar spine and increases wear on the feet, knees, and sacroiliac joints, all of which puts your back in danger. Instead, the obvious back-friendly choice are comfortable, low-heeled shoes.

Backache R$_x$

If you already have back pain, don't despair, because there are many helpful options available to you. Ice helps control swelling and muscle spasms in the early stages (about the first three days); after that, moist heat helps increase circulation and mobility. Also, consider visiting a chiropractor for spinal manipulation and alignment.

Bed rest is the wrong response to back pain (as if your baby would

allow that anyway!). Research shows that staying active is very important in treating or controlling back pain. Counterirritants, such as cap-
saicin cream (made from spicy cayenne peppers), applied topically help
control back pain.[4]

BENIGN BREAST PROBLEMS

Tender breasts that feel lumpy are the characteristic symptoms of fibrocystic breast disease, a condition that varies in intensity throughout the
menstrual cycle. Supplemental intake of one of the following nutrients
might relieve the symptoms of fibrocystic breast disease: vitamin E (400
IU), vitamin B_6 (10–25 mg), evening primrose oil (3 grams), and vitex
(40 drops of a concentrated extract).

If you have breast pain or fibrocystic breast changes (especially if
your breast pain feels achy and dull in one or both breasts), you might
consider avoiding caffeine. Compounds called methylxanthines, which
are found in caffeinated coffee and tea (even chocolate to a degree),
might promote the formation of painful breast cysts. It may take one to
two months of being caffeine-free for the pain to decrease or go away
completely.

BREAST CANCER

In the 1950s, one American woman in twenty was at risk for developing breast cancer. Today, one in eight is at risk, and about forty thousand women die as a result of it annually.

What you put on your dinner plate plays a major role in breast
cancer risk. In fact, 38 percent of breast cancers in the United States
could be prevented by dietary changes. The basic nutrition message here
won't be surprising at all: aim for a balanced diet consisting of plenty
of fruits, vegetables, and whole grains. Try to get five servings of fruits
and veggies each day, select whole grains (as opposed to refined ones),
eat less fat and sugar, and focus on calcium-rich foods. In addition, take
a daily multivitamin with folic acid.

Fiber doesn't just help keep you regular, it may also lessen your

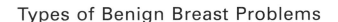

Types of Benign Breast Problems

Most women probably will experience a lump, growth, cyst, or pain in their breast sometime in their life. Among the most common:

- **Cyst:** A harmless, fluid-filled sac that may develop in the breast, a cyst may feel tender and even painful.

- **Fibroadenoma:** A solid, painless lump. These lumps are not cancerous, but they may get bigger during pregnancy and breast-feeding.

- **Fibrocystic breast changes:** A generalized "lumpiness" to the breast tissue; this is so common that it is now considered to be a variation of normal for breasts. The symptoms of lumpiness, discomfort, a heavy feeling, and tenderness may vary from mild to severe and also change throughout the menstrual cycle. Fibrocystic breast changes do *not* increase the risk of breast cancer.

- **Infection or inflammation:** This is most common in breast-feeding women, as a result of a blocked milk duct or a bacterial infection. It is uncommon in women who aren't nursing. An infection sometimes develops when sebaceous material around the nipple becomes infected.

- **Mastalgia:** Breast pain ranging from minor to severe, this often cycles with a woman's period.

- **Nipple discharge:** For non–breast-feeding women, the most common time to experience nipple discharge is near menopause. It may be caused by a blocked breast duct or a wartlike growth (called a papilloma) in a duct near the nipple, or it may be associated with cancer.

chances of developing breast cancer. Women should aim for 28 grams of fiber daily (the average American gets just 10–15 grams).

Fiber-rich foods include whole grains, nuts, fruits, and vegetables— foods that should sound familiar, since they are the same ones that form the basis of a healthy, anticancer diet in general. Fiber keeps breast cancer at bay, especially in premenopausal women, by clearing out excess estrogen.[5] Fiber also indirectly fights cancer by helping you keep your

Breast Cancer Risk Factors

There are numerous factors that raise your risk of developing breast cancer, including:

- Family history of breast cancer

- Onset of menstruation before age 12

- Beginning menopause at a late age

- Giving birth after age 30 to your first child

- Never giving birth

- Being 40 percent above normal weight for your age and height

weight in check;[6] studies clearly show that being overweight is a big risk factor for breast cancer.

Soy foods (as well as a handful of other foods, such as flax seeds, sesame seeds, lentils, and whole-grain cereals) contain phytoestrogens, which are estrogen-like compounds found in plants. Since breast cancer has a hormone component, many women feel confused as to whether they should include soy in their diet or avoid it.

Some cancer experts feel that the concerns about soy have been overstated. In short, soy does not cause breast cancer. The research is very consistent that if soy is eaten from a young age and throughout life, it is associated with lowering the risk of breast cancer. But here's the big caveat: those who have been diagnosed with breast cancer may not want to eat soy daily or take soy-based supplements.

Traditional Asian soy-based foods (such as tofu, miso, and natto) are certainly healthy and safe in moderation, meaning two to four servings a week; however, highly processed and concentrated forms of soy, such as isoflavone supplements, do not have the same clear safety record.

Consider pouring yourself a cup of green tea every day. When researchers took a close look at the beverage choices of thousands of women (both with and without breast cancer), they found that women who regularly drank green tea had a 12 percent lower risk of developing breast cancer. The more years and the more often these women drank green tea, the stronger was their protection from breast cancer.[7]

Alcohol in any form (even wine!) ups the chance of breast cancer. Just one drink a day will increase your lifetime risk of breast cancer by 5 percent, and it goes up from there (with six daily drinks raising your risk by a whopping 40 percent).

It seems that alcohol affects the way that the body handles estrogens (and this is particularly true for the synthetic estrogens in hormone therapy), with the end result being an increase in estrogen's influence on cancer. As a double whammy, alcohol saps the body of the B vitamin folic acid. Folic acid plays a key role in producing new body cells, and it also guards against DNA changes that lead to cancer. When alcohol reduces the body's folic acid supply, this cancer watchdog is no longer on guard against breast cells that could become cancerous.

Breast Self-Exams: What to Look For

Regular breast self-exams and an annual clinical exam from your gynecologist can identify many breast problems in the early stages. If you notice any of the following symptoms in your breasts, contact your doctor right away:

- A lump, hard knot, or thickening
- Swelling
- Redness
- Warmth
- Change in size or shape
- Skin dimpling or puckering
- Rash
- Spontaneous nipple discharge (not related to lactation)

Note: It's normal to experience breast tenderness around ovulation.

When it comes to alcohol, the best advice for those concerned about breast cancer is to drink less. But if you do drink, supplement with folic acid for some extra protection.

BREAST-FEEDING CONCERNS

Numerous books and resources contain information about and help in establishing the breast-feeding relationship. I am not going to duplicate that work, but will cover a few issues connected to lactation and alternative medicine.

First, it's a good idea to keep taking your prenatal vitamin/mineral supplement while nursing. Another very helpful supplement to continue using after pregnancy is omega-3 fatty acids, since they contain docosahexaenoic acid (DHA), which is very important for healthy development of the brain and eyes of infants. DHA passes from the mother's diet into breast milk.

Several herbs are known as galactagogues, which means that they encourage milk production. These herbs, which include fenugreek, stinging nettle, vitex, and goat's rue, have a rich history of common use in the European herbal tradition. Experts disagree as to whether vitex is helpful during lactation, with some evidence indicating increased lactation and other evidence showing decreased lactation.[8]

For sore nipples, applying a warm, moist poultice made with soothing herbs such as chickweed and comfrey to the affected breast may soothe the irritated tissue. (Wash the breast before nursing.)

COLDS AND THE FLU

The average American comes down with two to four colds each year. Add kids to the mix and the numbers go even higher. But you don't have to be one of the statistics. There are effective ways to sidestep the next bug making the rounds in your community.

Regular, moderate exercise primes the immune system to be efficient and effective, but too much exercise may be too much of a good thing. Prolonged and intense training, such as running marathons, is taxing to many parts of the body, including the immune system. Immunity may be impaired for several days after strenuous exercise. You'll definitely want to fit in some regular exercise, but now may not be the best time to train for a marathon.

Stress—whether physical, emotional, or mental—is a major drain on immunity. Incorporating stress management into your daily life is a great way to keep immunity on track, while having the added benefit of making you feel better overall. Granted, this is particularly difficult advice for new parents, since the first year of a new baby's life adds a lot of unavoidable stress. Just do the best you can here.

Vitamin C has long been linked to the common cold, and with good reason. There is some evidence that it may also be helpful for those stricken by the flu. People under stress appear to gain the most benefit from this cold-fighter.[9] Taking 500 mg of vitamin C daily makes colds less frequent, according to a five-year-long study published by Japanese researchers.[10] If you've neglected to take a daily supplement of vitamin C but feel your throat start to tickle, the earlier you reach for the bottle of vitamin C supplements, the more likely it is that you'll stave off a cold. Try 3–5 grams of vitamin C daily in divided doses during a cold; if this amount triggers GI upset, take less.

The mineral zinc, in lozenge form, is another powerful weapon for keeping cold viruses from gaining a foothold in your respiratory tract.[11] Colds get better more quickly and the symptoms are less severe in those sucking on zinc lozenges every couple of waking hours. Dissolve a zinc lozenge in your mouth every two to three waking hours for the duration of your cold.

Vitamin D makes the body more effective at killing bacteria and viruses that would otherwise trigger an infection. The majority of adults run low on this vitamin (due to wearing sunscreen faithfully and valid concerns about avoiding too much sun exposure). Supplemental vitamin D makes sense; aim for 400–1,000 IU daily.

Elderberry extract is another great option during a cold or flu attack. It seems to work most effectively when its use is started within twenty-four hours of the first symptom.

Andrographis, also known as Indian echinacea, has been used for

Germ-Fighting Habits

Follow these simple tips to keep nasty germs at bay and stay healthier:

1. The best way to prevent the spread of disease is one of the easiest and most straightforward: wash your hands. Banish bugs by sudsing and scrubbing for at least 20 seconds after using the bathroom, after diaper changes, before eating, and especially after being around ill people.

2. Maintain moist mucous membranes—which physically block the entrance of viruses through the nose, eyes, or mouth—by drinking plenty of water, wearing lip balm, and using a humidifier during the cold, dry season.

3. On a weekly basis, disinfect germy areas around the house, such as remote controls, phones, computer keyboards and mice, light switches, and doorknobs.

4. Get plenty of sleep each night to recharge your immune system—most people need seven to eight hours per night. As a new parent, this is the most challenging advice to follow, so just do the best you can.

the treatment of colds and flu in both Ayurvedic and Traditional Chinese Medicine because of its ability to stimulate the immune system. Modern scientific research confirms that this herb eases cold and flu symptoms.[12] Andrographis has a great safety record, however it can cause slight stomach upset in a small percentage of people; this might be avoided by taking it with food or lowering the dosage. Try 200 mg per day of a standardized extract of andrographis.

CONSTIPATION

Constipation is a common health complaint in the United States, and this problem may be especially vexing for women recovering from a tear or episiotomy, or those who had prolonged pushing with labor or hemorrhoids during pregnancy.

Constipation occurs when a person has a decrease in daily bowel movements and/or passes hard, dry stool. Pain or difficulty passing stool is common with this condition. Sadly, most people would never have to deal with a bout of constipation if they ate right. But the way things stand with the average American diet, an estimated 10 percent of us suffer from constipation. Keep in mind that constipation may be a sign of a disease, such as irritable bowel syndrome, diverticulitis, or hypothyroidism.

Simply increasing fiber in the diet will resolve constipation in most cases; look to fruit, vegetables, whole grains, and legumes, or even a high-fiber supplement. Women should aim for at least 28 grams of fiber daily. Keep in mind that any increase in high-fiber foods should be gradual to help prevent bloating and gas. As an added benefit, increasing fiber intake not only supports good digestion in terms of regularity and healthy bacteria in the colon, but also contributes to cardiovascular health, weight management, and blood pressure control.

Fiber keeps things moving through the intestine. In addition, fiber acts as a sponge, attracting water to the stool. This is why it's important to drink plenty of fluids, too—at least eight glasses a day. Increasing fiber intake without boosting fluids may backfire and make constipation worse. Without adequate fluids, stool becomes hard and may even develop rough edges, which may produce tiny tears in the rectum. Feel free to choose from a variety of water, juice, herbal tea, and soup, but avoid black and green teas, since they contain tannins that help bind stools. Prunes and prune juice are time-honored constipation remedies, and for good reason: they work.

Spending more time at the gym or even taking a simple walk around the neighborhood on occasion may help, since physical activity promotes a well-functioning bowel and stimulates the wavelike contractions of the intestines known as peristalsis.

Even if your diet is full of fiber and fluids, you may become constipated if you ignore the urge to have a bowel movement. Waiting allows more water to be absorbed by the large intestine, leading to harder stool that is painful to pass. To maintain regularity, take the time to go to the bathroom as soon as you feel the urge.

Herbal Laxatives

Psyllium, flaxseed, fenugreek, and glucomannan have a high fiber content that supplies extra bulk to the stool. They also contain mucilage, which expands when it comes in contact with water (that's why these laxatives *must* be taken with plenty of water). These herbs are fairly mild, bulk-forming laxatives that can be used on an ongoing basis, if desired. They generally lead to a bowel movement within twelve to twenty-four hours.

Herbal stimulants tend to be more potent than the bulk-forming herbs. Stimulant herbs, such as senna, cascara, aloe, and rhubarb, contain natural laxative compounds called anthraquinone glycoside that stimulate contractions of the bowel muscles. Of all the stimulant herbs, cascara and rhubarb are the mildest. Aloe may be very potent and should be used cautiously.

These stimulant laxative herbs should be a last resort, only after you've tried dietary changes and bulk-forming herbs. These herbs may also cause dependency (that is, your bowels won't move without them), so they should be used only for short periods to prevent dependency. Do not use these stimulant herbs if you are pregnant.

DIARRHEA

Episodes of loose watery stools that occur three or more times in one day are generally considered to be diarrhea. Abdominal cramps, nausea, vomiting, fever, loss of appetite, and bloody or foul-smelling stools are often present as well. Many serious diseases can cause diarrhea (including infections that continue to rank as a leading killer of children in developing countries), but this discussion is limited to the common, run-of-the-mill diarrhea bouts that tend to resolve themselves within forty-eight hours. Diarrhea lasting longer than this will need to be treated by a physician, rather than with at-home remedies.

The most important thing to do for diarrhea is to stay hydrated. Diarrhea causes the body to lose lots of fluids, and this risk of dehydration is the most common medical consequence of ordinary diarrhea. It cannot be emphasized strongly enough: during a bout of diarrhea, drink lots of water or other fluids.

The BRAT diet is also useful for an acute bout of diarrhea. *BRAT* stands for the mild, well-tolerated foods bananas, rice (white rice is preferable to brown rice), apples, and toast (usually low-fiber toast is best, so as not to aggravate the diarrhea). These foods provide nutrients, such as fiber and potassium, that help treat diarrhea.

As your diarrhea subsides, you'll want to continue to be gentle to your recovering intestines by eating a simple diet that is easily processed, such as soup, cereal, crackers, mashed potatoes, or other foods that seem appetizing to you during your recovery. For the next day or two, avoid dairy products, high-protein foods, and fatty foods.

Diarrhea Triggers

Some people are sensitive to coffee, and drinking several cups daily may induce diarrhea. If you're a coffee drinker and regularly have trouble with diarrhea, consider avoiding all coffee for a few days to see if there is an improvement in your bowel habits. Lactose intolerance (the inability to digest milk sugar) can cause diarrhea, as well as cramps and gas. Avoiding dairy products, switching to easier-to-digest ones (such as yogurt), or using a lactase supplement may resolve this problem.

A type of fruit sugar called sorbitol may trigger diarrhea in some sensitive people. Sorbitol is absorbed slowly, and during its stay in the intestine sorbitol tends to hold onto water, leading to diarrhea. If you suspect that you could be reacting to sorbitol, try avoiding it. Read labels on all the foods you eat, and don't eat foods with this ingredient, or fruit juice, to see if this simple change gets rid of your problem.

Taking too much of the dietary supplements vitamin C or magnesium may sometimes cause diarrhea. The amount that is problematic varies for each individual, and other signs of illness (such as fever) do not accompany the diarrhea in this case. More than a few grams per day of vitamin C are generally needed to initiate a problem; however, many people are not bothered by ten times this amount. For magnesium, most people do not have a problem until intake exceeds 350–500 mg per day. Keep in mind that magnesium-containing laxatives are a source of magnesium and taking too many of them for constipation may end up causing diarrhea.

Antibiotics have been a double-edged sword. Since their discovery, they have cured previously incurable diseases and saved countless lives. However, antibiotics kill the helpful bacteria along with the bad, leaving your intestinal tract devoid of its important friendly flora.

When the good bacteria that usually reside in the intestine are killed off, diarrhea often results. Replenishing supplies of beneficial bacteria is important after a course of antibiotics. Active-culture yogurt or supplements providing beneficial bacteria may also be taken as a preventive during antibiotic use. In fact, taking probiotic supplements to replace the beneficial bugs may cut in half your chances of antibiotic-induced diarrhea.

Probiotics, such as *Lactobacillus acidophilus* and bifidobacteria, replenish your body's "friendly bacteria" after a bout of diarrhea. Probiotics in food are found in various dairy products, chiefly yogurt, kefir (drinkable yogurt), cottage cheese, and a handful of fluid milk products. Check the label for which species of bacteria and how much of them are present, as products vary widely and you need billions of live cultures to replenish the good bacteria in your gut.

Herbal Diarrhea Remedies

Numerous herbs may be helpful in treating loose bowels. The antidiarrheal herbs generally contain one or more of three basic ingredients: tannin, pectin, or mucilage. Tannins are compounds in herbs that act as astringents. The astringency of tannins is the reason they lessen intestinal inflammation. Pectin adds bulk to stool because it is a soluble fiber. Mucilage also adds bulk, but it does this in a different way—by absorbing water and swelling in size. Mucilage also soothes the digestive tract.

Carob is a prime example of an herb that provides tannins. Carob may be used for adult cases of diarrhea, as well as cases that occur in children or infants. Other astringent herbs include blackberry and red raspberry. The leaves of these two herbs can be used to make an astringent tea. Bilberry, in the form of dried berries or juice, also provides tannins, but the fresh berries should not be used because they may worsen diarrhea. Both green tea and black tea are very astringent and fit the bill for a beverage of choice during diarrhea.

Mucilage-providing herbs include marshmallow and slippery elm. These may be very soothing to the digestive tract. Fenugreek seeds are another rich source of mucilage, but they should be limited to two teaspoons (10 ml) at a time; otherwise, they may induce abdominal distress.

FIBROIDS

Uterine fibroids, medically known as leiomyoma or myoma, are classified as benign since they are noncancerous. They generally crop up within the muscle layer beneath the endometrium (the lining that sheds monthly) and are composed of fibrous material—hence the common name *fibroids*. A woman might only have one fibroid, but they tend to grow in clusters—ranging from the size of a pea to the size of a grapefruit.

For something that doctors call "benign," fibroids sure can cause a lot of pain and turn your life upside down. One in four women has difficulties with fibroids—and an even greater number of women have fibroids that are asymptomatic.

Fibroids tend to strike women during the prime of life—and in the prime reproductive years—causing the hallmark symptoms of heavy, painful periods. Severe menstrual cramps, backache, frequent urination, intense PMS, constipation, hemorrhoids, urinary urgency, painful intercourse, and even infertility are also associated with fibroids.

Fibroids are more responsive to estrogen than normal muscle tissue. Basically, this means that estrogen prompts them to grow bigger. Thus, during times of higher estrogen secretion, such as pregnancy, or when taking estrogen-containing birth control pills, they can mushroom rapidly. And it follows, then, that they tend to shrink away after menopause, when estrogen levels in the body naturally decline.

Naturally, if your fibroids do not cause you any discomfort, you can simply do nothing aside from regular pelvic exams to monitor their growth. In addition, since menopause generally signals the end of fibroids, some women who have mild cases of fibroids or are close to menopause opt for the path of "watchful waiting." Watchful waiting does not mean that you have to suffer in silence. There are several natural ways to treat the discomforts caused by fibroids.

Because fibroids are associated with estrogen levels that are out of whack, there are a lot of things you can do to get back into hormone balance; this should then hopefully lead to a lessening of fibroid symptoms. Regular exercise is a great way to lower circulating levels of estrogen, along with providing myriad other health perks.

The connection between estrogen levels and exercise is well-known; however, there have not yet been any scientific studies to test whether starting an exercise regimen will actually resolve symptoms in women with uterine fibroids. Aside from the ovaries, fat cells are the leading producers of the hormone estrogen. Women with greater stores of body fat have higher estrogen levels, and a higher risk of fibroids goes hand in hand with the spike in estrogen. Eating a higher-fat diet also adversely influences estrogen levels. Choosing a lower-fat diet, along with a sensible exercise program, should lead to weight loss, and the combination of these factors may have a dramatic, beneficial effect on estrogen.

Consider dabbling in vegetarianism. When the diets of women with fibroids were compared to those without, a few differences stood out as significant. First, fibroid sufferers ate more beef, other red meats, and ham. Second, green vegetables and fruit were conspicuously absent from their plates. All the fiber in a vegetarian-style diet is part of the answer. A fiber-packed diet helps shuttle extra estrogen out of the body.

What do you do with the hole left on your dinner plate once meat is booted out (at least for some of the meals)? Consider soy. The consumption of soy foods, such as tofu, tempeh, and soy milk, alters estrogen production and metabolism; the net result is a lowering of circulating estrogen. Several servings of soy foods daily would be needed to positively alter estrogen levels. One serving equals one cup (200 ml) of soy milk or one-fourth of a block of tofu. A small number of people are allergic to soy; do not consume soy products if you're allergic to soy.

The roles of the hormones estrogen and progesterone are intertwined. The herb vitex sparks the body's production of progesterone to correct hormone imbalances.[13] Take note, however, that vitex is not quick-acting; it may take several months to yield a benefit. Do not consume vitex during pregnancy, since there is a slight concern that this herb (by encouraging menstruation) could interfere with pregnancy.

The liver is ground zero when it comes to metabolizing and excreting estrogen. It follows, then, that a healthier liver gives you a better chance of maintaining balanced hormone levels. Drinking alcohol and eating heavy, fatty foods puts a lot of stress on the liver and should therefore be minimized. Milk thistle is best known as a liver-friendly herb. Compounds in milk thistle, called silymarin, protect the liver in many ways, such as blocking the entrance of toxins into the liver, boosting antioxidant defenses in the liver, and even regenerating damaged liver cells. Try a supplement providing 250 mg of silymarin per day. Milk thistle may have a mild laxative effect in some people for the first few days of use.

Who's at Risk for Uterine Fibroids?

Women with the following risk factors are more likely to develop fibroids:

- Thirty-five to 50 years old (although fibroids may occur in women as young as 20 years old).
- Never been pregnant.
- Currently pregnant (if fibroids are already present, they grow faster during pregnancy).
- Taking high-dose-estrogen birth control pills.
- Overweight, especially "apple"-shaped body type.
- Have female relatives with fibroids.
- Under high amount of stress (either physical or emotional).
- African-American (3–9 times more likely to have fibroids than Caucasian women).
- A history of using an IUD that caused infection.
- Use of talc powder around the vulva.

The heavy bleeding that many women with fibroids experience may deplete iron stores and cause anemia. Anemia, in turn, saps your life energy, leaving you feeling drained, run-down, and foggy-headed. If this sounds like you, it's a good idea to have a blood test to check your iron status. Good food sources of iron include organ meats, dried fruits, beans and peas, and blackstrap molasses. Iron supplements may be needed for those with anemia, perhaps up to 100 mg per day, but should only be taken by those diagnosed with anemia. Many multivitamin/mineral supplements contain a much lower amount of iron (generally 18 mg) that may help prevent a deficiency from developing in the first place.

FIBROMYALGIA

If you're a woman in your early thirties and experience chronic muscle pain, stiffness, and trouble sleeping, you're not alone. You may be one of the 3 million to 6 million people suffering from fibromyalgia. There is a lot that doctors don't understand about fibromyalgia—such as what causes this complex disorder, or what cures it. What *is* known is that many of those suffering from fibromyalgia are women twenty-five to forty-five years old. These women (and men, too) report the primary symptoms of aches and pains in their muscles, tendons, and ligaments. Other common symptoms include fatigue, swelling, muscle spasms, stiffness, headache, and difficulty getting a good night's sleep. There is a possibility that fibromyalgia is hereditary.

Since the symptoms of fibromyalgia are somewhat vague, misdiagnosis is common. Cases of fibromyalgia are often misdiagnosed as hypothyroidism, rheumatoid arthritis, chronic fatigue syndrome, lupus, or other disorders. Although fibromyalgia generally emerges between the ages of twenty-nine and thirty-seven years of age, most people are not correctly diagnosed until the ages of thirty-four to fifty-three years old—with the intervening years often spent being treated for one of the above-mentioned misdiagnosed conditions.

Until a cure is found, treatment for fibromyalgia focuses on easing the symptoms of this syndrome with nutrients or therapies to manage pain, improve sleep quality, and increase energy levels. A good place to start is an examination of the overall diet—you should be eating adequate amounts of all the essential vitamins and minerals. Caffeine, alcohol, and nicotine should be avoided, since they interfere with sleep and energy patterns.

Several studies involving patients with fibromyalgia suggest that a combination supplement providing magnesium and malic acid may relieve muscle pain. After taking 300–600 mg of magnesium and 1,200–2,400 mg of malic acid each day for eight weeks, the individuals in these studies reported significant pain relief. The B vitamin thiamine may also be involved in fibromyalgia, since some studies have found fibromyalgia patients to have low thiamine status. However, the exact role that this vitamin might play in the onset and ongoing symptoms of fibromyalgia remains unclear.

Exercise is among the most important recommendations for people with fibromyalgia. Start out with low-impact aerobic exercise, such as swimming, stationary bicycling, or walking, for as little as a few minutes every other day, and build up to twenty-minute sessions three to four times a week. Once you feel comfortable with a regular exercise regimen, more intense exercises, such as jogging or tennis, may be incorporated. Since stress may exacerbate symptoms of fibromyalgia, stress reduction techniques, such as meditation, may also be helpful.

FOOT PROBLEMS

Many women find that their feet get bigger during pregnancy; mine certainly did. I grew a half-size. Perhaps the biggest annoyance stemming from this pregnancy effect is the potential to have to get rid of a lot of great shoes. The extra water your body holds onto during pregnancy can cause swollen feet, and that will go away after your baby is born. If your feet are still bigger now than before your pregnancy, it is due to pregnancy hormones that caused the ligaments in your feet to relax, resulting in slightly wider feet. These changes, I'm sorry to say, are permanent.

Eight out of ten women report experiencing minor but troubling foot ailments, such as blisters, corns, ingrown nails, and heel pain. In most cases, a little attention could put the spring back in your step. Even something as simple as over-the-counter shoe inserts, called orthotics, may greatly improve foot comfort. OTC orthotics are a great value for women who have mild heel pain, although they may not be the best choice for someone with severe pain or a deformity that has been present for a long time. However, a woman who has metatarsalgia (pain in the ball of the foot) when wearing heels, may find comfort in an orthotic designed to wear in heels, for instance.

Shoe-Shopping Tips

1. Feet tend to swell during the day, so try on shoes at the end of the day, when your feet are at their largest.

2. Most women haven't had their feet measured in years (you might be surprised to find out that your size isn't what you think it is!). Measure your feet, and do it while you're standing up for the most accurate reading.

3. Choose a shoe that's designed with a leather upper, a stiff heel counter, appropriate cushioning, and flexibility at the ball of the foot.

4. Check that the shoe fits well—front, back, and sides—to best distribute weight.

5. Make sure shoes don't pinch your toes, either at the tips, or across the toe box; if so, put them back (no matter how cute they are!).

6. Always try on both shoes, and walk around the store.

7. Make sure that the shoe fits your larger foot (almost everyone has one foot that's a bit larger than the other).

8. Don't buy shoes that need a "break-in" period; shoes should be comfortable immediately.

9. Wear the socks or stockings you'll be wearing with this shoe to make sure everything feels comfortable together.

10. If you wear orthotics or shoe inserts, take them along when you try on shoes.

GAS

Everyone has gas. Burping or passing gas is normal, but because it is embarrassing or uncomfortable, many people worry that they have an abnormal amount. The average person will pass gas more than a dozen times a day, most of which isn't noticed. It's only when excessive amounts of gas build up, leading to a bloated, painful feeling, or when the gas is malodorous, that it becomes problematic. Most of the time gas is odorless. The odor comes from sulfur made by bacteria in the large intestine. In addition to the digestive process, air may be swallowed while eating or drinking and add to the amount of gas in the intestinal tract.

Certain foods are notorious gas producers. Beans and legumes, in particular, cause foul-smelling gas for many people. Soaking beans overnight and then discarding this water before cooking them may remove some of the indigestible sugars in beans that produce gas during digestion.

Gas-forming foods also include cauliflower, broccoli, Brussels sprouts, cucumbers, red and green peppers, and onions. Fiber-rich foods may also be problematic in this regard. Gradually increasing the fiber content of your diet should keep this to a minimum, however.

Lactose intolerance may be a major reason a person is plagued with gas, as well as cramps and diarrhea. While avoiding dairy products will eradicate this source of gas, total avoidance may not be necessary; many people with lactose intolerance can eat small amounts of dairy products, particularly yogurt. Another option is to take supplements of lactase—the enzyme needed to digest lactose—right before a meal that contains dairy products.

Including active-culture yogurt in your diet may help normalize the bacterial residents in your intestinal tract and minimize gas. Supplements of the probiotic acidophilus achieve the same effect.

There are a few short-term solutions for reducing gas, including charcoal tablets that absorb gas and digestive enzymes (if inadequate stomach acid or lactose intolerance is your problem). If you try charcoal, do not be surprised if your stools temporarily turn black.

Antigas Tips

- Eat smaller portions.

- Chew food thoroughly.

- Sip, rather than gulp, liquids.

- Avoid carbonated beverages.

- Do not chew gum.

- Do not drink with a straw.

- Remain in an upright position while eating.

- The product Beano contains natural enzymes that reduce gas when it is used along with troublesome foods.

A class of herbs called carminatives work to quell excessive gas and ease painful spasms in the intestinal tract. Peppermint, fennel, and caraway are premiere members of this class. Used alone or in combination, these herbs have been found in several studies to reduce gas and cramping.

HAY FEVER (SEASONAL ALLERGIES)

If you are wary of taking OTC or prescription medications while nursing, but suffer from hay fever, you might want to consider some natural remedies. However, keep in mind that these natural remedies, while helpful, are not going to give you the same relief as conventional medications.

During an allergy attack, proteins called histamines start roaming the body, producing itchy eyes, a drippy nose, sneezing, headaches, and a whole array of other symptoms that plague nasal passages, eyes, throat, lungs, skin, and even the digestive tract. A natural antihistamine, vitamin C, blocks the release of histamine and gets rid of histamine that's already making the rounds. For best effect, vitamin C (1–2 grams) and quercetin (500–1,000 mg) need to be taken daily starting several weeks prior to allergy season.

Quercetin is a plant pigment found especially in apples, onions, and black tea. Like vitamin C, quercetin is a natural antihistamine that counteracts the body's excessive histamine release during an allergy attack. It does this by strengthening cell membranes so any histamine in the cell is less likely to leak out into surrounding tissues. As an added bonus, quercetin also dampens inflammation, which may congest allergic nasal

Anti-Allergy Tips

- Try to stay mostly indoors during peak pollen season, especially on dry, windy days.

- When pollen counts are high, wash bedding regularly and bathe before bedtime, so pollens stuck to your hair and skin don't irritate you while you sleep.

- Consider using a neti pot (a small pot with a spout that is used to irrigate the nasal passages) to flush out allergens.

- Eating fresh produce and whole grains, and cutting out refined sugar, may reduce flare-ups and minimize symptoms.

- Shut your closet doors. Sounds simple, but it helps because it keeps your clothes away from the dust mites that may trigger indoor allergies. If outdoor allergens bug you, avoid hanging laundry outdoors.

- Plan outdoor activities for lower-pollen days.

- Avoid mowing the lawn; but if you can't, wear a surgical mask to limit your exposure to pollens.

- Avoid cigarette smoke and other respiratory irritants.

- If you're sensitive to animal dander, keep pets out of your bedroom or even out of the house entirely.

- If you're sensitive to dust mites, use plastic or vinyl covers over pillows and mattresses.

passages. Start taking quercetin as soon as allergies hit, and keep using it daily throughout allergy season. To be on the safe side, quercetin should not be used during pregnancy because of an isolated test tube study suggesting that this supplement could encourage cell mutations.

Thymus extracts come from thymus glands (most often from young calves); they help to get your own thymus gland working better. Perched in the chest below the thyroid and above the heart, this butterfly-shaped gland is a serious immune-system player, pumping out infection-fighting white blood cells called T-lymphocytes. Thymus extracts seem to balance the immune system. During hay fever and other allergy flare-ups, the immune system overreacts to pollen, animal dander, mold, and the like, mistakenly attacking them as if they were dangerous infectious agents. According to older research, taking a thymus extract daily reduces the number of allergy attacks and eases allergy symptoms.[14]

HEADACHES (NONMIGRAINE)

Tension headaches create steady, nonthrobbing pain that feels like a tightening band around your forehead and extends down your neck; these headaches account for about 90 percent of all headaches. Triggers for these run-of-the-mill headaches include things that new parents are very familiar with, such as too little sleep and being overwhelmed by stress. Anxiety and depression may also serve as tension headache triggers.

The good news is that you can make changes to your diet and lifestyle that have a good chance of helping you sidestep some of your headaches. The bad news is that it may be a bit tricky to figure out which things are triggers for you, since different things serve as headache triggers for different people. Certain food components in cheese, chocolate, red wine, beer, and processed meats, as well as MSG, aspartame, caffeine, sulfites, and tartrazine (FD&C yellow #5), are among the more likely headache precipitators. Getting too little sleep, not drinking enough water, and allowing your stress level to rise may also bring on head pain.

Keeping a headache diary will help you pinpoint which foods or lifestyle choices are behind your pain. To speed up the process, you might want to cut out the most common food triggers listed above. Add them back one by one and note any headaches that occur afterward. Symptoms may appear as long as three days after consuming one of these trigger foods, so it can be tricky to identify your headache culprit. Caffeine may be a double-edged sword when it comes to headaches. Consuming caffeine causes headaches in some susceptible people, yet for others who consume caffeine on a regular basis, skipping a coffee break may lead to a caffeine-withdrawal headache.

Willow bark is recommended for the relief of run-of-the-mill headaches. Willow is often referred to as "herbal aspirin," since aspirin was created from its active ingredient. The pain-relieving actions of willow are typically slow-acting but last longer than standard aspirin products. As with aspirin, long-term use of willow may cause stomach irritation and should not be used by children or individuals allergic to aspirin.

You can also try peppermint oil. Applying a 10 percent peppermint oil solution to your temples during a headache might help you feel better.

HEADACHES (MIGRAINE)

Women are three times as likely as men to be the unfortunate recipient of a migraine, probably because of a hormonal factor involved in migraines. Food allergies, birth control pills, and stress may all trigger migraines. In addition, there seems to be a genetic component to migraines. While OTC pain relievers help ease the pain of a migraine, many people with migraines end up needing a prescription medication to treat an attack.

Migraines are an intense headache that may last from a few hours to a few days. The pain is often one-sided, described as throbbing or pulsating, and accompanied by nausea and vomiting and sensitivity to light. Migraines are divided into two classes: the "classic" migraine is preceded by the warning sign of an aura (a visual disturbance) before the headache strikes, while the "common" migraine lacks this warning aura.

Profiles of Headaches

Caffeine withdrawal headache: Regular users of caffeine may develop throbbing headaches twelve to twenty-four hours after abstaining from caffeine. The headache goes away if caffeine is consumed or withdrawal symptoms will resolve themselves within two to seven days on their own.

Cluster headache: Cluster headaches concentrate most of the pain around one eye, have a rapid onset, and recur in clustered groups for days, weeks, or months until a remission period. Smoking is a risk factor for these headaches and they are more common in men.

Dehydration headache: Dehydration may trigger a headache, which is easy to remedy by simply drinking water.

Eyestrain headache: Too much computer work may trigger a headache. Resting your eyes several times an hour and possibly getting prescription glasses geared toward computer use may solve the problem.

Ice cream headache: A short-lived, but intense, pain that generally follows the ingestion of ice cream (or other cold foods and beverages). About one-third of the population is susceptible to "brain freeze." This condition resolves itself quickly and doesn't require any treatment (except for the obvious and difficult-to-follow advice to eat ice cream more slowly).

Migraine headache: The "classic" migraine is an intense, throbbing headache (lasting from hours to days) accompanied by nausea and vomiting and preceded by the warning sign of an aura (visual disturbance). The "common" migraine has the same symptoms, but without the visual disturbances.

Rebound headache: Taking acetaminophen, ibuprofen, or aspirin too often may actually result in a "medication overuse" or rebound headache. Avoid this trouble by limiting analgesic use to no more than twice a week.

Sinus headache: This refers to a headache that develops as a result of a sinus infection. The pain is centered around the eyes and cheeks, and worsens when bending over. These headaches are actually rare; many supposed cases of sinus headache are actually migraines.

Tension headache: This type of headache—the old vise grip around the temples—is the most common form of headache and causes a sense of fullness or pressure in the scalp, the forehead, and the back of the neck.

Thunderclap headache: A sudden and severe headache, often described as the worst headache possible, could signal a life-threatening condition, such as a stroke or an aneurysm. Seek immediate medical attention.

The herb feverfew may ease the frequency, severity, and length of migraine attacks. Although scientists aren't certain exactly how feverfew works to prevent migraines, several studies show that taking this herb daily protects against migraines.[15] Choose a feverfew product that supplies at least 250 mcg of parthenolides per day. Remember: while this herb may make migraines less frequent and less severe, it is not useful to start taking it once a migraine sets in. Instead, you need to take it daily as a preventive. Do not take this herb if you're pregnant or breast-feeding, since there is a lack of safety data with this herb during these times.

Levels of the mineral magnesium tend to be lower in people with recurrent migraines. When people suffering from frequent migraines participated in a study supplementing them with 600 mg of magnesium daily for three months, they reported a significant (42 percent) drop in the frequency of their migraines.[16] Keep in mind that the high amount of magnesium used in most research studies—600 mg daily—may cause diarrhea. If that occurs, try magnesium in the form of magnesium citrate or lower your dosage to 200–300 mg and see if you still benefit without the GI upset.

So-called "menstrual migraines" may strike each month around the time of a woman's period (as a result of falling estrogen levels). Taking magnesium every day for a week or two prior to your period's arrival (300 mg in the morning and 300 mg in the evening) may help you sidestep this type of headache. Again, if this amount of magnesium causes GI trouble, try a lower dose or the more gentle magnesium citrate form.

A supplement called coenzyme Q_{10} may keep migraines at bay if taken every day. When a group of forty-two migraine sufferers did just that, they had fewer migraines; in fact, almost half of them slashed in half the number of days with migraine (compared to placebo).[17] If you want to try this for yourself, you'll need to take 150–300 mg daily. (But be forewarned: this is a pricey supplement.)

HEMORRHOIDS

Hemorrhoids are one of the most common ailments known, with more than half the population experiencing them at some point in life. Hemorrhoids are varicose veins that occur in the anus and rectum. In general, they are the result of excessive pressure on the veins in that area. They are more common with advancing age, during pregnancy, and if you have a family history of hemorrhoids, experience frequent constipation or diarrhea, or overuse laxatives or enemas.

Hemorrhoids are classified as either internal or external, depending on their location. External hemorrhoids feel like a hard lump and are very sensitive. Internal hemorrhoids may protrude during bowel movements, which may or may not be painful. Other symptoms of hemorrhoids are itching in the anal area or bleeding during bowel movements.

The straining that accompanies constipation places extra pressure on the affected veins, either causing or worsening hemorrhoids. Therefore, treating underlying constipation is an important first step for resolving hemorrhoids.

People who have a high fiber intake are less likely to develop hemorrhoids. Remember to drink more fluids any time you eat more fiber. The insoluble form of fiber, which is primarily found in whole grains and vegetables, makes the stool softer, bulkier, and easier to pass. Supplementary fibers, such as psyllium seeds, may also be used to increase fiber intake.

In the meantime, sitting in a warm sitz bath may help relieve the pain and itching of hemorrhoids. The herb witch hazel has astringent properties that may help shrink hemorrhoids. It can be applied as an ointment to the affected area a few times a day. A gel containing the herbal extract horse chestnut may be used for the same purpose.

Vitamin C and a class of nutrients called bioflavonoids help heal and strengthen blood vessels. Eating more fruits and vegetables to up your fiber intake will naturally provide more of these nutrients as well. They are also available as supplements.

INDIGESTION

If you ever get that vague feeling of abdominal discomfort, often coupled with heartburn, upset stomach, bloating, or gas, you're not alone. About half of us endure indigestion every so often, and an unhappy 25 million Americans face it daily.

The cause of indigestion is often a mystery, although there are certainly factors that can make it more likely, including obesity, pregnancy, medications (such as aspirin, oral contraceptives, and certain antibiotics), eating too much, eating too quickly, or eating while you're under too much stress.

A wholesome, low-fat diet goes a long way toward digestive health. Ditch fatty foods, which lead to indigestion, since they take longer to digest and result in a full, bloated feeling, and even pain. Foods and beverages (including coffee, tea, colas, and tomato-based foods) that crank up acid in the stomach should be avoided, or at least minimized, if they are a problem for your tummy. Alcohol and tobacco are also promoters of sour stomach. Other changes that may prevent indigestion include the following: eat smaller meals at regular intervals, don't exercise on a full stomach, and don't lie down within two hours of eating.

If prevention didn't pan out and your stomach is still churning, then chamomile is your go-to herb. Chamomile is good for stomach ailments of all sorts, including indigestion; it soothes an irritated digestive tract and encourages normal digestion. The tea form is particularly comforting.

Another good bet is licorice (the herb, not the candy). Licorice protects the mucous membranes that line the digestive tract against the damaging effects of stomach acid. This effect is particularly helpful for those with heartburn. Licorice root extract in the form of deglycyrrhizinated licorice (DGL) is preferable, since the glycyrrhizin component of licorice may cause high blood pressure. Try one to two chewable DGL tablets (250–500 mg per tablet) fifteen minutes before meals and one to two hours before bedtime. Do not take licorice during pregnancy as there is a slight risk of miscarriage or early delivery.

Bitter herbs encourage salivation and production of stomach acid and digestive enzymes—in other words, they get your juices flowing. There are many herbs with bitter properties, but gentian is one of those used most often for this purpose. Others include dandelion, bitter orange, centaury, and blessed thistle. Bitters are particularly valuable for people who eat a lot of fatty, hard-to-digest foods. One or more of these bitter herbs may be used by adding approximately 2 ml of tincture (concentrated liquid extract) to a glass of water and sipping it before a meal. Do not use these if you have ulcers or gastritis.

For some people, indigestion results from the body not making enough pancreatic enzymes (which are important during the digestive process). Certain medical tests can assess the body's production of digestive enzymes. An easier way is to simply add digestive enzymes to a meal and see if your digestion improves. Try 500 mg of bromelain, 25–50 mg of papaya enzyme, or, for pancreatic enzymes, follow the label directions.

For years, it was assumed that taking digestive enzymes before a meal was best. But all this changed now that researchers in Spain finally put this assumption to the test and found that taking the enzymes before a meal was actually the least effective mode of ingestion.[18] So take digestive enzymes during a meal or at the completion of a meal.

IRRITABLE BOWEL SYNDROME

Irritable bowel syndrome (IBS) is characterized by crampy pain, bloating, gas, and altered bowel habits. People with IBS often alternate between constipation and diarrhea. It is not known what causes IBS, and it has proved difficult to treat with conventional medicine. For some people, IBS is just a mild annoyance, but for others it is disabling since they can never be far from a bathroom.

Although stress was once thought of as the cause of IBS, it is now known that emotional conflict and stress do not cause the disease. Stress does, however, worsen symptoms. Many people report more intense symptoms of IBS while under stress. Relaxation techniques or counseling help relieve IBS symptoms in some people.

Although there is no specific "IBS diet" that will work for everyone, individualized changes to your diet may be very helpful. This means doing a bit of sleuthing to see if any particular foods trigger your symptoms. Food triggers may include chocolate, dairy products, sorbitol, alcohol, and caffeine.

Dietary fiber is helpful to many people with IBS.[19] By including high-fiber foods in your diet, such as whole-grain breads and cereals, beans, fruits and vegetables, or a supplement, such as psyllium, the bowels become more regular, with fewer bouts of constipation. Go slowly if you're increasing your fiber intake; adding too much too quickly may cause gas and bloating—which are among the symptoms you are trying to eliminate. Also, while you gradually up your fiber intake, make sure you also increase your fluids (at least eight glasses of water a day). Without this extra water, you could end up with hard stools that are painful to pass.

Not all fibers are equal, however. Wheat bran as a source of fiber has been reported in some research to make people with IBS feel worse, which may indicate that wheat allergy is common in IBS.

Several herbal remedies offer relief from IBS symptoms. Peppermint helps because it lessens the production of gas, eases intestinal cramps, and soothes irritated tissues. Most research uses the enteric-coated capsule form of peppermint oil, which ensures that the oil is released in the intestines instead of the stomach.[20] Start with one capsule (0.2 ml per capsule) of enteric-coated peppermint three times a day, in between meals (swallow, don't chew, the capsules!). If you experience a burning sensation when you move your bowels, then switch to just two pills a day, or even just one pill daily. The Indian spice turmeric (500 mg four times per day) and slippery elm powder (follow label directions) may also help soothe an irritated GI tract.

OSTEOPOROSIS

Osteoporosis is a preventable disease in many cases if optimal calcium intake is maintained throughout life. Plenty of calcium during childhood and the teenage years is important for building strong, dense bones. During the middle years of life, optimal calcium intake slows the natural loss of calcium from the bones. And, in later years, especially for women after menopause, calcium intake may prevent the rapid bone loss associated with the advanced stages of osteoporosis.

There is more calcium in the human body than any other mineral. And 99 percent of the 1,200 grams of calcium found in the average body is contained in bone tissue. Adult women are advised to get 1,000 mg of calcium every day. Optimal calcium intake before age twenty-five is crucial for building strong, osteoporosis-resistant bones, but it's never too late to reap the benefits of calcium.

Calcium-rich foods are a no-brainer when it comes to building better bones. Dairy products are a dependable source of calcium, as are leafy-green vegetables (such as collards, kale, and parsley), sea vegetables (such as kelp and dulse), broccoli, and tofu. There are also a few no-no's when planning an osteoporosis-resistant diet: skip the saltshaker, cut back on caffeine, and avoid soft drinks that contain phosphoric acid.

Vitamin D is also important, since it is needed to absorb calcium, as well as to prevent demineralization of the skeleton. Vitamin D helps your body turn calcium into bone. Although human skin can synthesize vitamin D when exposed to sunlight, as a result of geography, clothing choices, or staying inside, many people simply don't produce enough of this vitamin. Vitamin D is underappreciated for its crucial role in preventing osteoporosis. Vitamin D is vital for getting calcium into the body and keeping it in the bones. Strong bones require adequate vitamin D.

Exercise is another key player. Weight-bearing exercise, such as walking, jogging, aerobics, dancing, and stair climbing, slows the loss of bone. As little as thirty minutes per day can make a difference.

THYROID PROBLEMS

Thyroid problems are common in women who have had a baby recently. It is easy to overlook or rationalize the symptoms of low thyroid function (hypothyroidism), since so many symptoms of hypothyroidism mimic what new moms generally experience: fatigue, depression, constipation, headache, dry skin, hair loss, and an inability to lose weight.

Don't underestimate the importance of the thyroid gland, since this little butterfly-shaped gland nestled below your throat pretty much rules your body. The thyroid gland serves as a thermostat for metabolism, so an underactive thyroid (hypothyroidism) slows the body down, while an overactive thyroid (hyperthyroidism) revs everything up.

Hypothyroidism—by far the more common form of thyroid problem—crops up more often in women with advancing age and in those with a family history of thyroid problems. There's quite the laundry list of potential symptoms with hypothyroidism: fatigue, forgetfulness, depression, heavier periods, dry hair and skin, mood swings, weight gain, intolerance to cold, hoarse voice, and constipation. If you suspect a problem with your thyroid, ask your doctor for a blood test to assess your thyroid hormone levels. If your levels run low, thyroid hormones will likely be needed to make up the difference, but there are a few things you can do nutritionally to support a healthy thyroid.

The mineral selenium, in the form of selenium methionine, is essential to the conversion of thyroid hormone into its active form, which is why taking 200 mcg of this mineral daily may be helpful. If you don't want to take a supplement, you also can get this amount of selenium from one big handful of Brazil nuts (by far, the best food source of the mineral).

Zinc is another mineral that is essential to the thyroid hormone pathway, conversion, and production process. Taking 10 mg of zinc daily supports thyroid function, and it's a good idea to add in 1–2 mg of copper daily (to counteract zinc's action of blocking copper absorption).

The amino acid L-tyrosine is necessary to manufacture thyroid hormone. Too little L-tyrosine in the body limits the amount of thyroid hormone that the body can make. So supplements of L-tyrosine can kick-start sluggish thyroid conditions. However, supplementing with L-tyrosine may be too stimulating to some people, so it's advisable to start with a lower dose (200 mg or less per day) and work up to a maximum of 500 mg, as long as no side effects are noted. This amino acid has a tendency to increase blood pressure, so you may want to skip this supplement if high blood pressure is a concern.

Iodine is an essential nutrient, as well as an ingredient in making thyroid hormone. But iodine may be tricky, because while iodine deficiency is a major thyroid risk factor, too much iodine may aggravate the thyroid, cause thyroid enlargement (called goiter), and worsen existing thyroid conditions. Certainly there's no harm for anyone with thyroid concerns to include iodine-rich foods in the diet, such as seafood and seaweed (kelp and bladderwrack are great choices). But unless you're tested as iodine-deficient, you probably shouldn't supplement with this mineral.

URGE INCONTINENCE

Urge incontinence—also known as overactive bladder—causes a sudden, overwhelming need to urinate, as well as urine leakage in some cases. It's much more common in women than men, especially after becoming a mom.

Several years ago, researchers studying the benefits of magnesium supplements for women with calf-muscle spasms accidentally discovered that this mineral seems to also help with urge incontinence. Double-blind research followed, showing that magnesium does, in fact, help some women with urge incontinence.

Kegel exercises may improve bladder problems like urinary frequency, urgency, urge incontinence, and stress-related urinary incontinence. Pelvic-floor exercises work for both prevention and treatment, and you only need to set aside five to ten minutes every day or so. Women with the goal of preventing bladder problems should do them for a shorter time less often, and those with an active problem would best be served by more frequent, longer exercise sessions. However, it may take up to two months of exercising the pelvic floor before a woman

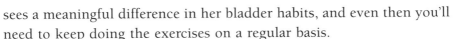

sees a meaningful difference in her bladder habits, and even then you'll need to keep doing the exercises on a regular basis.

Before you start, you need to find the right muscles. Here's a simple trick: stop your stream when urinating (but don't do this all the time since it could actually cause a voiding problem); the muscles you are tightening to do this are the pelvic floor muscles—the ones to put to work in the following exercises.

Quick flick: For this exercise, contract and release the pelvic-floor muscles quickly in a series of ten or more. Just as with any new exercise program, these exercises could leave you tired or even sore, so start out with a few series, and slowly work your way up.

Long hold: Start by contracting and holding your pelvic-floor muscles for as long as you can; this will show your baseline strength. To do the actual exercise, contract and hold for half of your maximum time and rest for that same amount of time. So if your maximum hold was eight seconds, your exercise will start with four-second holds, alternating with a four-second rest. Repeat ten times, and when it feels easy, increase your hold times.

URINARY TRACT INFECTIONS

Urinary tract infections (UTIs) are an uncomfortable and frequent annoyance for many women. Bladder infections start when bacteria, most often *Escherichia coli,* migrate up the urethra and start growing in the bladder. The female anatomy (specifically, a shorter urethra) provides an easier route for bacteria to infect the bladder than the male anatomy, which is a primary reason that far more women than men develop UTIs. A common scenario is for a woman to develop several UTIs a year, take antibiotics each time to treat the UTI, and subsequently come down with a secondary yeast infection because of the antibiotics and then need to treat *that* infection. And on it goes. As if that weren't enough trouble, UTIs increase the risk of kidney infections.

Eight out of ten women will experience a UTI at least once in their life and 20 percent of women develop a UTI annually. And once a woman has experienced a UTI, her risk of recurrence is a whopping 20–30 percent. The infection usually goes like this: bacteria migrate from the GI tract to the urinary tract and adhere to the mucosal cells along the urinary tract. This is the critical first step in the development of a UTI. Stop the bacterial adherence and you stop an infection.

Cranberry juice was first put to the scientific test in the early 1900s. Back then, researchers suspected that the acidity of cranberry juice somehow made the bladder inhospitable to the bacteria that cause UTIs. Since that time, however, researchers discovered that cranberries inhibit the growth of UTI-causing bacteria in a totally different way than was first suspected. This tart fruit contains compounds called proantho-cyanidins that block bacteria from sticking to the bladder walls, thereby derailing a budding infection. Simply put: if the bacteria can't attach, then they can't start trouble as an infection before being washed away in the urine.[21]

The power of cranberries to eradicate urinary tract infections is astounding: recurrence of UTIs are slashed in half when women either drink cranberry juice or take tablets of cranberry juice extract. In a study of women plagued by recurrent bladder infections (a disheartening six or more in the prior year), supplementing with cranberry extract brought that number to zero, and women who continued supplement-ing remained infection-free during the next two years.[22]

When researchers compared antibiotics head to head with daily sup-plements of cranberry extract, it turned out that both treatments had nearly the same effectiveness in keeping UTIs at bay.[23] Although antibi-otics were slightly better in this regard than cranberry, cranberry gets bonus points for not causing the many downsides of antibiotics; that is, diarrhea, stomach upset, yeast infection, or even potentially fatal superinfections. Remember, though, that cranberry is about prevention; it doesn't help treat an active infection.

While cranberry juice and tablets of cranberry juice extract are both effective choices for preventing UTIs, don't rely on cranberry juice "cocktails," since these are heavily sweetened and contain only a very small amount of cranberry juice.

For women who find that bladder infections keep popping up, pro-

UTI Prevention Tips

All women (especially those with a propensity to recurrent UTIs) should take these additional steps to reduce the risk of UTI:

- Drink plenty of fluids.

- Void regularly (especially after sexual activity).

- Wipe from front to back.

- Avoid the use of diaphragms and spermicides.

- Wear cotton underwear.

biotic bacteria offer some hope. Research shows that several strains of the bacteria *Lactobacillus* reduce the chances of developing a bladder infection. *Lactobacillus* bacteria grow in colonies. Large colonies of these helpful bacteria form a barrier that physically bar *E. coli* and other harmful bacteria from migrating into the bladder, where they would otherwise cause an infection.[24] Supplementing with *Lactobacillus* (1–10 billion live organisms daily) or regularly including fermented dairy products in your diet (such as yogurt, kefir, cottage cheese, and some fluid milk products) will lessen the chances of developing a UTI.

YEAST INFECTION

Yeast infections caused by an overgrowth of the fungus *Candida albicans* are most common in the vagina, and factors that can alter the vaginal environment and precipitate an overgrowth of the fungus include pregnancy, diabetes, menstruation, douching, feminine hygiene sprays, oral contraceptives, and antibiotics.

The telltale signs of yeast infection include itching, a white discharge, irritation, redness, swelling, and soreness during intercourse. Of course, any woman who is unsure about whether her symptoms are a yeast infection should see her doctor for a diagnosis.

Friendly bacteria, also called probiotics, keep the *Candida* fungus in check to both prevent and treat yeast infections. Acidophilus, when applied topically, eaten as active-culture yogurt, or taken as an oral supplement, has been found by scientific research to prevent vaginal yeast infections.

When women who had a history of recurrent yeast infections followed a daily regimen of consuming eight ounces (227 g) of yogurt (with active acidophilus cultures) daily for six months, they reported a threefold reduction in the number of yeast infections during the study period.[25] Studies involving the topical application of yogurt have shown similar benefits.

APPENDIX

Herb and Dietary Supplement Safety

Even if there is a long history of safe use for the majority of herbal remedies consumed today, most herbs and dietary supplements have not been thoroughly researched with human clinical trials when it comes to use during pregnancy and lactation. As such, the data regarding safety during pregnancy and lactation is incomplete. This appendix compiles information from the limited research that is available, but keep in mind that herbs may have powerful properties, and some caution is necessary. Watch your baby closely for any adverse reactions if you take any herb or medicine while nursing.

5-HTP. There are some reports of nausea with 5-HTP. There are some anecdotal reports of vivid dreams (and even nightmares) from taking large amounts of 5-HTP. People taking antidepressants (including SSRIs and MAO inhibitors) should not take 5-HTP.

7-Keto. Research is too limited (and there is no history of use) to establish safety of this supplement during pregnancy or lactation.

Acetyl-L-carnitine. Side effects are rare, but skin rash and body odor have been reported.

Aloe. Aloe taken orally (as opposed to topically) may be very potent and should be used cautiously. Use only for short periods to prevent bowel dependency. Do not use while pregnant or breast-feeding.

Alpha-lipoic acid. There are rare reports of mild stomach upset or allergic skin rash from this supplement.

Andrographis. This herb may cause slight stomach upset in a few people, which might be avoided by taking it with food or lowering the dosage. Safety in pregnancy and nursing is unknown.

Arginine. If you suffer from bouts of cold sores or genital herpes, you shouldn't take arginine because it may stimulate the virus that causes those conditions.

Arnica. For topical use only. Arnica may cause itching and rash in sensitive individuals.

Ashwagandha. No known side effects.

B-complex vitamins. Take B-complex vitamins with food to prevent queasiness that may result otherwise.

Bee pollen. There are rare reports of allergic reactions.

Beta-carotene. At very high doses, this may cause a harmless (and reversible) yellow coloring in the palms of the hands and the soles of the feet.

Bilberry. No side effects or cautions reported.

Biotin. No side effects or cautions reported.

Bitter herbs (gentian, dandelion, bitter orange, centaury, and blessed thistle). These should not be used by anyone with ulcers or gastritis.

Black cohosh. Both the British Herbal Pharmacopoeia and the American Herbal Products Association caution against the use of black cohosh during pregnancy.[1]

Blackberry. There are reports of nausea in some sensitive individuals.

Bloodroot. Do not use if you're pregnant or nursing.

Borage oil. Do not use while nursing.

Boswellia. Rare side effects include diarrhea, nausea, and skin rash.

Bromelain. Allergic reaction (rash, hives, breathing problems) has been reported, but it is extremely rare.

Butcher's broom. This herb is very safe.

Butterbur. Select a product that is labeled as containing no pyrrolizidine alkaloids (compounds that can cause liver damage).

Calcium. In individuals prone to kidney stones, calcium may raise the risk of stone formation. Some people report constipation, bloating, or gas when taking calcium supplements.

Caraway. Caraway is generally safe, although caraway oil should not be taken by pregnant women.

Carob. This herb is very safe, aside from very rare reports of allergic reactions (such as hives).

Carotenoids. This supplement is very safe.

Cascara. Do not use cascara if you're pregnant or nursing.

Cayenne (topical). Cayenne cream causes a mild burning feeling. Be sure to wash your hands after applying it and do not rub your eyes before washing.

Chamomile. Although very rare, allergic side effects (such as itching, rashes, and breathing problems) have been reported. This herb is considered safe for both pregnant and lactating women.

Charcoal. Charcoal temporarily and harmlessly turns the stools black.

Chasteberry. See *Vitex*.

Chickweed. No known side effects for the topical use of this herb.

Chitosan. Do not take this during pregnancy.

Chondroitin. No side effects reported, aside from nausea at very high intakes.

Chromium. Skin rash with this supplement is possible, but very rare.

Citicoline. Research is too limited (and there is no history of its use) to establish safety of this supplement during pregnancy or lactation.

Coenzyme Q_{10}. People with cardiomyopathy should not discontinue use of coenzyme Q_{10} without the involvement of a physician, since the condition may quickly worsen. Coenzyme Q_{10} should not be taken by anyone on warfarin because this supplement could decrease the effectiveness of the medication.

Coleus forskohlii. This herb should not be taken by anyone with ulcers. The safety in pregnant and breast-feeding women is unknown.

Conjugated linoleic acid (CLA). Rare side effect of GI upset has been reported. Breast-feeding moms shouldn't use CLA because it has been shown to lower the fat content of breast milk.

Copper. People with Wilson's disease should not take copper, since that disease prevents the body from getting rid of extra copper.

Cranberry juice extract. According to a handful of case reports, cranberry could increase the activity of warfarin.[2] Until more is known about this, anyone on warfarin should not use cranberry. Cranberry is considered safe during pregnancy and lactation.[3]

Curcurmin. People with gallstones should not take this herb. High amounts during pregnancy could, in theory, trigger contractions (although there are no reports of this happening before), but nonetheless it would be prudent to avoid this herb during pregnancy.

Damiana. No significant side effects, aside from a mild laxative effect at very high doses, have been reported. Do not take while pregnant.

Dong quai. Dong quai is not associated with side effects. Due to a lack of evidence of safety, it should not be used during pregnancy or lactation.

Elderberry. No side effects reported.

Epimedium. No significant side effects have been reported.

Fennel. Allergic reactions, such as hives and breathing problems, have been reported in rare cases.

Fenugreek. This herb may impart a harmless maplelike odor to sweat, milk, and urine of the woman taking it, as well as her infant if she's nursing.[4] Allergic reactions, such as hives or breathing difficulties, may occur in those allergic to chickpeas.

Feverfew. Minor side effects of GI upset reported in some people. Do not take feverfew while pregnant or breast-feeding.

Flax. Allergic reactions are very rare.

Folic acid. Do not take more than 1,000 mcg per day of folic acid since greater amounts may hinder the laboratory diagnosis of vitamin B_{12} deficiency.

Ginkgo. Very rarely, mild stomach upset and headaches are reported with ginkgo use. However, do not use if you take MAO inhibitors (a type of antidepressant). Do not use during pregnancy or lactation.[5]

Ginseng. Ginseng may cause headache, insomnia, palpitations, and a rise in blood pressure, if overused. Ginseng should not be taken by people with high blood pressure, diabetes (unless you work with your physician to adjust your insulin levels), or anyone taking MAO-inhibitor antidepressants or blood-thinning drugs. Ginseng is not recommended for pregnant or nursing women.

Glucomannan. This herb is generally safe.

Glucosamine. There are rare reports of GI upset with this supplement.

Goat's rue. This herb is considered generally safe during breast-feeding, although there is a report of two cases of infants experiencing drowsiness, lethargy, vomiting, and poor suckling when their mothers drank a goat's rue tea (containing goat's rue along with licorice, fennel, and anise).[6]

Gotu kola. No known side effects.

Green foods. Green foods are safe and beneficial for almost anyone (even during pregnancy). The only people who should avoid green foods are those with autoimmune diseases.

Green tea. This herb contains caffeine, and for that reason, may not be appropriate during pregnancy or nursing.

Guarana. This herb contains caffeine, and for that reason, may not be appropriate during pregnancy or nursing.

HCA. The compound HCA, extracted from *Garcinia cambogia* and *Garcinia indica* fruits, should not be taken while pregnant or nursing.

Hemp. Hemp can cause loose stools in a small number of people.

Hoodia. No side effects or cautions reported.

Hops. There are no side effects reported with this herb.

Horse chestnut. Rare cases of itching and nausea have been reported.

Huperzine. There are a few reports of dizziness with this herb.

Hyaluronic acid. This supplement can cause skin rash in rare cases.

Inositol. This supplement could theoretically stimulate uterine contractions, so it should not be used during pregnancy.

Iodine. Only people who have been tested and found to be iodine-deficient should supplement with this mineral.

Iron. Do not take a stand-alone iron supplement (which generally provides much more iron than a daily multi) unless a doctor has prescribed it. The potential for harm is greatest for older men and postmenopausal women, and both of these groups generally should *not* supplement with this mineral. Most people will suffer stomach upset and constipation from too much iron before any other adverse effects set in. People with hemochromatosis or hepatitis C should not supplement with iron.

Kola nut. This herb contains caffeine, so the same cautions of ingesting caffeine apply.

Lactase. No side effects reported.

L-carnitine. Higher amounts could cause diarrhea; extremely high doses can cause an unpleasant fishy body odor. Only L-carnitine should be used; the D, L-carnitine form may interfere with normal L-carnitine function in the body.

Lecithin. There are reports of people taking large amounts of choline (a source of lecithin) and experiencing GI upset and diarrhea, while extremely large amounts of choline can cause a fishy body odor and depression.

Licorice. Licorice root extract in the form of deglycyrrhizinated licorice (DGL) is preferable since the glycyrrhizin component of licorice can cause high blood pressure. Licorice should not be used during pregnancy.

L-theanine. There are no known side effects from this green tea extract.

L-tryptophan. This supplement shouldn't be used by anyone taking antidepressants and should also be avoided by those with cirrhosis. Dizziness and diarrhea have been reported occasionally. Do not use during pregnancy or lactation.

L-tyrosine. No significant side effects have been reported.

Maca. No significant side effects have been reported with this herb.

Magnesium. Higher intake of magnesium causes loose stools; this may happen with supplemental doses between 350 mg and 500 mg. People with kidney disease may have impaired ability to excrete extra magnesium from the body and for this reason should not supplement with magnesium.

Malic acid. No side effects or cautions reported.

Marshmallow. No significant side effects have been reported with this herb.

Melatonin. There are some reports of morning drowsiness with melatonin used for insomnia. Side effects with melatonin are infrequent, although people with epilepsy and those taking warfarin should not use melatonin. Due to a lack of data, it would be prudent for women who are pregnant or breast-feeding to not take melatonin.

Milk thistle. Milk thistle may have a mild laxative effect in some people for the first few days of use, but aside from that there are no known safety concerns and this herb is considered safe to use during pregnancy and lactation.[7]

Mucuna pruriens. Do not use this herb during pregnancy or lactation.

Muira puama. No safety concerns have emerged with *muira puama*, but due to a lack of safety data it would be prudent to avoid this herb during pregnancy and lactation.

Myrrh. No significant side effects have been reported with this herb.

Neem. Due to a lack of data, neem should be avoided during pregnancy.

Omega-3. Omega-3 fatty acids are safe during pregnancy and lactation.[8] They are well-tolerated, although some people experience upset stomach or "fishy" burps with the use of fish oils.

Pancreatic enzymes. This supplement should not be used by children with cystic fibrosis.

Papaya enzyme. Do not use during pregnancy, due to a slight risk of uterine contractions.

Passion flower. Do not use during pregnancy, due to a slight risk of uterine contractions.

Peppermint. This herb is generally safe, although it should not be used by people with chronic heartburn, liver damage, or gallstones.

Phosphatidylserine. There are no safety concerns with this supplement.

Proanthocyanidins. There are no safety concerns with this supplement.

Probiotics. There are no safety concerns with this supplement.

Psyllium. This herb is generally safe, although there have been some isolated reports of allergic reactions, such as hives and breathing problems.

Pycnogenol. There are no safety concerns with this supplement.

Pyruvate. Large amounts may trigger stomach upset, bloating, gas, and diarrhea in some people.

Quercetin. This supplement appears to be free of side effects; however, due to an isolated test tube study with bacteria, to be on the safe side this supplement should not be used during pregnancy.

Raspberry. This herb is considered safe for pregnancy and lactation, although it may cause slight bowel loosening.

Rhodiola. There are no reports of side effects with this herb.

Royal jelly. Royal jelly may trigger allergic reactions, such as hives and breathing problems, and it could adversely interact with the blood-thinning drug warfarin.

Sage. This herb should not be used during pregnancy.

Schisandra. There are rare reports of GI upset and skin rash with this herb.

Selenium. Taking too much selenium may cause garlic breath, hair loss, skin rashes, and brittle fingernails.

Senna. Use of this herb needs to be limited to no more than ten days or the bowel may become dependent on it. Do not use it if you have Crohn's disease, ulcerative colitis, or intestinal obstructions. The use of this herb during pregnancy and breast-feeding is controversial; it would be prudent not to use it.

Silicon. This mineral is not associated with any side effects.

Slippery elm. There are no side effects or cautions reported with this herb.

St. John's wort. This herb makes the skin more sensitive to sunlight, so rashes or burns may develop after sun exposure. There is not enough research to confirm the safety of this herb during pregnancy, although its use in lactation appears to be of minimal risk (with the caveat that there are a few cases reported of colic, drowsiness, or lethargy in the nursing infant).[9]

Stinging nettle. There are a few reports of mild stomach upset in some people and rare reports of allergic reactions, such as a rash. This herb is considered safe during pregnancy and lactation.

Tea tree oil. Tea tree oil is for external use only. It may irritate sensitive skin and some people are allergic to it. Apply a small amount to your inner arm as a test before you use tea tree oil; if your arm becomes red or inflamed, discontinue use.

Thymus extracts. There are no side effects reported with this supplement.

Turmeric. This herb may not be appropriate for people with gallstones. Although this herb has a long history of use during pregnancy, there is a theoretical risk of uterine contractions and for this reason it may be better to avoid during pregnancy.

Valerian. There are no reports of side effects or safety concerns with this herb.

Vinpocetine. There are no safety concerns with this supplement.

Vitamin B$_3$. The niacin form of vitamin B$_3$ can cause flushing, headache, and stomachaches, although these problems are unlikely with the sustained-release niacin. Unfortunately, this form of niacin can cause liver toxicity. The niacinamide form of vitamin B$_3$ is not associated with side effects.

Vitamin B$_6$. Do not take more than 200 mg of vitamin B$_6$ daily. Over time, high doses of vitamin B$_6$ may cause nerve damage, such as a tingling sensation in the hands and feet. It is safe during pregnancy and lactation in moderate dosages.

Vitamin B$_{12}$. There are no side effects associated with this supplement.

Vitamin C. The safety profile of vitamin C is outstanding, however, people with hemochromatosis (an iron-overload disease) shouldn't have extra vitamin C, nor should those susceptible to kidney stones. For anyone, higher doses of vitamin C (3–5 grams) may cause stomach upset and diarrhea.

Vitamin D. This supplement should not be taken by people with hyperparathyroidism.

Vitamin E. This supplement is safe at a wide range of intakes.

Vitex. The cautious course of action with this herb is to discontinue use if you become pregnant and do not take it if you're nursing. However, experts disagree as to whether this herb is problematic during lactation, with some evidence indicating increased lactation and other evidence showing decreased lactation.[10]

White-bean extract. There are some reports of diarrhea with the use of this herb.

Willow bark. As with aspirin, long-term use of willow could cause stomach irritation and should not be used by children or individuals allergic to aspirin.

Witch hazel. There are no concerns with the topical use of this herb.

Yellow dock. This herb has reportedly caused loose stools in some people.

Yerba mate. There is no safety data regarding pregnancy or lactation, so skipping this herb would be prudent.

Zinc. While moderate amounts of zinc support a healthy immune system, taking excessive amounts may have the opposite effect, increasing susceptibility to infections. However, even moderately high levels can cause nausea. *Note:* It's okay to take extra zinc for a short time, such as using zinc lozenges to treat the common cold.

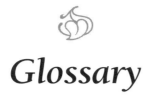

Glossary

Adaptogen: A category of herbs that have a balancing effect on the body and increase resistance to the damaging effects of stress.

Adrenal glands: Endocrine glands that produce adrenaline and other hormones.

Amino acids: The building blocks of protein.

Analgesic: A drug that reduces or takes away pain.

Anemia: Condition characterized by a reduced number of red blood cells; symptoms include fatigue, unclear thinking, and poor concentration.

Antibody: Protein produced by the immune system that recognizes and attaches to foreign substances. This makes it easier to destroy or eliminate the foreign substance, be it a toxin or a germ.

Antioxidant: A compound that neutralizes free radicals otherwise associated with degenerative diseases, such as cancer, heart disease, and premature aging.

Ayurveda: A traditional system of medicine practiced in India since the first century CE. Ayurvedic practitioners combine herbs, oils, and other natural systems in treating diseases. Many herbs used in Ayurveda are now gaining popularity in Western countries.

Baby blues: Feelings of anxiety and depression in the days or weeks after having a baby.

Bacteria: Single-celled microorganisms. Some cause disease, while others are harmless or even beneficial to biological processes.

Basal metabolic rate: Energy used for maintaining basic body processes, such as breathing and heartbeat.

Bile: Bitter-tasting fluid produced by the liver and stored in the gallbladder before being released into the small intestine to assist in the digestion of fats.

Bioflavonoids: A class of phytonutrients that have antioxidant, antibacterial, antiviral, and anti-allergenic properties.

Blood pressure: The forces placed on the blood vessels by the flow of blood.

Bone marrow: Soft material filling the inside of bone cavities; produces blood cells and platelets.

Bowel: Small or large intestine.

Caffeine: This chemical, which is present in tea, coffee, and chocolate, is a member of the family of chemicals called methylxanthines and acts as a central nervous system stimulant.

Cancer: General term for various illnesses characterized by abnormal growth of cells.

Capillaries: Tiny blood vessels connecting the smallest arteries to the smallest veins.

Carbohydrate: Compounds composed of starches or sugars. Bread is an example.

Carcinogen: Potential cancer-causing agent.

Cardiovascular disease: Diseases affecting the heart and blood vessels, including coronary artery disease and hypertension (also known as high blood pressure).

Caries: Decay of teeth due to bacteria; also known as cavities.

Cavity: An area of the tooth where the enamel has been destroyed by bacterial plaque.

Cervical dysplasia: A precancerous condition of the cervix.

Cholesterol: A fatlike substance found in foods and produced by the liver. High levels circulating in the blood are a risk factor for cardiovascular disease.

Collagen: A protein comprising connective tissues.

Colon: The large intestine, extending from the small intestine to the anus.

Constipation: The difficult passage of hard, dry stools.

Dementia: Mental deterioration leading to the inability to think clearly or function normally.

Deoxyribonucleic acid (DNA): A substance found in the nucleus of cells that carries genetic information.

Detoxification: Process of cleansing the body of drugs and other toxins.

Diabetes: A disorder characterized by high levels of glucose in the blood. It may be caused by a failure of the pancreas to produce sufficient insulin or by resistance of the body to the action of insulin.

Double blind: A type of research study in which neither the researchers nor the subjects know who's getting the medicine and who's getting the placebo until the code is broken at the end of the study.

Edema: Swelling of body tissues due to excessive fluid.

Electrolyte: A substance or salt that dissolves into positive- or negative-charged particles and conducts an electrical charge; sodium, potassium, and chloride are examples.

Enamel: The hard, calcified outer layer of the teeth.

Endocrine: The system of glands in the body that secrete hormones.

Endometriosis: A health condition in which a woman experiences considerable pain, cramping, and heavy bleeding during menstruation.

Endorphins: Proteins that create positive feelings in the body.

Enzyme: A complex protein present in digestive juices or within cells that acts as a catalyst for chemical reactions.

Ergogenic aid: Any substance that improves athletic performance.

Estrogen: One of the hormones produced by a woman's body that governs many body processes.

Feces: Body waste discharged from the bowels.

Fibrocystic breast disease: An umbrella term for any condition of the breasts causing painful lumps.

Fibroids: Noncancerous lumps that grow in the uterus.

Free radicals: Highly reactive compounds that damage cell membranes and other cell components, contributing to degenerative diseases, such as heart disease, cancer, premature aging, cataracts, and many other conditions. They are found in air pollution, tobacco smoke, some foods, pesticides, and ultraviolet radiation. They are also manufactured during normal body processes.

Galactagogues: Herbs that encourage or support milk production.

Gallbladder: Sac located under the liver; stores bile secreted by the liver.

Gastrointestinal (GI) tract: The digestive system structures, including the stomach and the intestines.

Gingivitis: Inflammation of the dental gums; the beginning stage of periodontal disease.

Glucose: Another word for *sugar*, often used in reference to blood sugar.

Glycogen: A storage form of glucose in the body. The liver produces glycogen from glucose and the muscles can use it as energy.

Heart attack: Myocardial infarction, the technical term for a heart attack, occurs when the blood flow to the heart is severely limited or stopped.

Hemochromatosis: A disorder that causes too much iron to be stored in the body.

Hypertension: Blood pressure readings above 140/90 are considered high and indicate that the heart and arteries are under excessive strain. Also known as high blood pressure.

Hyperthyroidism: A condition in which the thyroid gland produces excessive amounts of thyroid hormone.

Hypothyroidism: A condition in which the thyroid gland produces too little thyroid hormone.

Immune system: The body's resistance to disease that is provided by many specialized organs, tissues, and chemicals working together.

Influenza: A viral infection causing symptoms similar to those of the common cold, but more serious. Severe cases may lead to life-threatening complications and even death.

Insulin: A hormone produced by the pancreas that regulates blood sugar levels.

Isoflavone: Compounds in soy (genistein, daidzein, and glycitein) that have estrogenlike and antioxidant activity.

Kidneys: The two bean-shaped organs responsible for the excretion of urine and the regulation of water and electrolytes.

Lignan: One of the three main classes of phytoestrogens. Flaxseed oil and whole grains are rich sources of lignans.

Liver: An important organ that secretes bile, detoxifies the body, and stores glycogen.

Microorganisms: Bacteria, viruses, and other minute life forms that are only visible through a microscope. Many of these cause infections.

Minerals: Inorganic substances, such as calcium and magnesium; many are essential for health.

Mitochondria: Structures found in all cells that are responsible for producing energy.

Neural tube defects: Birth defects, such as spina bifida or anencephaly, caused when the embryonic neural tube that forms the future brain and spinal column fails to close properly.

Neurotransmitter: A hormonelike chemical that helps nerve cells communicate with each other or with muscles and organs.

Obesity: Body weight in excess of 20 percent above ideal body weight.

Oral: Pertaining to the mouth.

Osteoporosis: A condition involving porous, brittle bones that are prone to fractures.

Oxidation: Free radical damage to cells, tissues, and organs; associated with an increased risk of heart disease, cancer, and other degenerative diseases.

Pancreas: An organ in the abdomen responsible for producing and secreting several digestive enzymes and the hormone insulin.

Periodontal disease: Serious dental condition in which the gums are inflamed and may recede from the tooth and teeth may loosen.

Phytoestrogen: Plant compounds that have estrogenlike activity in the body.

Phytonutrient: Nonnutritive, but health-enhancing compounds derived from many plant sources.

Placebo: An inactive medicine or pill containing no active ingredients.

Placebo-controlled: Referring to a study in which a group of volunteers gets a medicine and another group, called the control, gets a dummy pill.

Plaque: A deposit of bacteria and other material that may build up on tooth surfaces, leading to tooth decay. Also, refers to deposits of cholesterols that build up along blood vessel walls.

Postpartum: The time just after giving birth.

Postpartum depression: Clinical depression that may affect some women after having a baby.

Premenstrual syndrome (PMS): A combination of physical and emotional symptoms occurring a week or two prior to menstruation.

Serotonin: A brain chemical that plays a role in mood.

Thymus gland: A gland in the chest that participates in the production of white blood cells.

Tonic: An herb that increases energy levels and feelings of vitality.

Tumor: An abnormal growth of tissue; it may be cancerous or noncancerous.

Thyroid gland: A gland in the throat that affects metabolism.

Ultraviolet (UV) radiation: A range of wavelength radiation present in sunlight. Excessive exposure to this damages and ages the skin.

Virus: A tiny organism that causes disease.

Vitamins: Essential nutrients found in foods, required in minute amounts but absolutely essential to the body. There are two classes of vitamins: water-soluble, such as vitamin C, and fat-soluble such as vitamin E.

References

Chapter 1. Losing the Baby Weight

1. Klem, M. L.; Wing, R. R.; Lang, W.; et al. Does weight loss maintenance become easier over time? *Obesity Research* 2000; 8 (6): 438–444.

2. Maki, K. C.; Reeves, M.S.; Farmer, M.; et al. Green tea catechin consumption enhances exercise-induced abdominal fat loss in overweight and obese adults. *Journal of Nutrition* 2009; 139 (2): 264–270.

3. Zenk, J. L.; Frestedt, J. L.; and Kuskowski, M. A. HUM5007, a novel combination of thermogenic compounds, and 3-acetyl-7-oxo-dehydroepiandrosterone: each increases the resting metabolic rate of overweight adults. *Journal of Nutritonal Biochemistry* 2007; 18 (9): 629–634.

4. Preuss, H. G. *Citrus aurantium* as a thermogenic, weight-reduction replacement for ephedra: an overview. *Journal of Medicine* 2002; 33 (1–4): 247–264.

5. Heiss, C. J.; Shaw, S. E.; and Carothers, L. Association of calcium intake and adiposity in postmenopausal women. *Journal of the American College of Nutrition* 2008; 27 (2): 260–266.

6. Kaats, G. R.; Michalek, J. E.; and Preuss, H.G. Evaluating efficacy of a chitosan product using a double-blinded, placebo-controlled protocol. *Journal of the American College of Nutrition* 2006; 25 (5): 389–394.

7. Kelley, D. S., and Erickson, K. L. Modulation of body composition and immune cell functions by conjugated linoleic acid in humans and animal models: benefits vs. risks. *Lipids* 2003; 38 (4): 377–386.

8. Blankson, H.; Stakkestad, J. A.; Fagertun, H.; et al. Conjugated linoleic acid reduces body fat mass in overweight and obese humans. *Journal of Nutrition* 2000; 130: 2943–2948.

9. Masters, N.; McGuire, M. A.; Beerman, K. A.; et al. Maternal supplementation with CLA decreases milk fat in humans. *Lipids* 2002; 37 (2): 133–138.

10. Roongpisuthipong, C.; Kantawan, R.; and Roongpisuthipong, W. Reduction of adipose tissue and body weight: effect of water soluble calcium hydroxycitrate in *Garcinia atroviridis* on the short term treatment of obese women in Thailand. *Asia Pacific Journal of Clinical Nutrition* 2007; 16 (1): 25–29.

11. Tominaga, Y.; Mae, T.; Kitano, M.; et al. Licorice flavonoid oil effects body weight loss by reduction of body fat mass in overweight subjects. *Journal of Health Science* 2006; 52 (6): 672–683.

12. Lenz, T. L., and Hamilton, W. R. Supplemental products used for weight loss. *Journal of the American Pharmacological Association* 2004; 44 (1): 59–67.

13. Kremer, R.; Campbell, P. P.; Reinhardt, T.; et al. Vitamin D status and its relationship to body fat, final height, and peak bone mass in young women. *Journal of Clinical Endocrinology Metabolism* 2009; 94 (1): 67–73.

14. Celleno, L.; Tolaini, M. V.; D'Amore, A.; et al. A dietary supplement containing standardized *Phaseolus vulgaris* extract influences body composition of overweight men and women. *International Journal of Medical Science* 2007; 4: 45–52.

15. Andersen, T., and Fogh, J. Weight loss and delayed gastric emptying following a South American herbal preparation in overweight patients. *Journal of Human Nutrition and Diet* 2001; 14 (3): 243–250.

Chapter 2. Kitchen Table Woes

1. Mattes, R. D., and Popkin, B. M. Nonnutritive sweetener consumption in humans: effects on appetite and food intake and their putative mechanisms. *American Journal of Clinical Nutrition* 2009; 89 (1): 1–14.

2. Bleich, S. N.; Wang, Y. C.; Wang, Y.; et al. Increasing consumption of sugar-sweetened beverages among US adults: 1988–1994 to 1999–2004. *American Journal of Clinical Nutrition* 2009; 89 (1): 372–381.

Chapter 3. Supercharge Your Nutrition

1. Muller, H.; Lindman, A. S.; Blomfeldt, A.; et al. A diet rich in coconut oil reduces diurnal postprandial variations in circulating tissue plasminogen activator antigen and fasting lipoprotein (a) compared with a diet rich in unsaturated fat in women. *Journal of Nutrition* 2003; 133 (11): 3422–3427.

2. Leung, B. M., and Kaplan, B. J. Perinatal depression: prevalence, risks, and the nutrition link—a review of the literature. *Journal of the American Dietetic Association* 2009; 109 (9): 1566–1575.

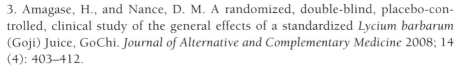

3. Amagase, H., and Nance, D. M. A randomized, double-blind, placebo-controlled, clinical study of the general effects of a standardized *Lycium barbarum* (Goji) Juice, GoChi. *Journal of Alternative and Complementary Medicine* 2008; 14 (4): 403–412.

4. Landrigan, P. J.; Claudio, L.; Markowitz, S. B.; et al. Pesticides and inner-city children: exposures, risks, and prevention. *Environmental Health Perspectives* 1999; 107 (S3): 431–437.

5. Mendola, P.; Selevan, S. G.; Gutter, S.; et al. Environmental factors associated with a spectrum of neurodevelopmental deficits. *Mental Retardation and Developmental Disabilities Research Reviews* 2002; 8 (3): 188–197.

6. Guillette, E. A. A broad-based evaluation of pesticide-exposed children. *Central European Journal of Public Health* 2000; 8 (Suppl): 58–59.

7. Guillette, E. A.; Meza, M. M.; Aquilar, M. G.; et al. An anthropological approach to the evaluation of preschool children exposed to pesticides in Mexico. *Environmental Health Perspectives* 1998; 106 (6): 347–353.

8. Asami, D. K.; Hong, Y.; Barrett, D. M.; et al. Comparison of the total phenolic and ascorbic acid content of freeze-dried and air-dried marionberry, strawberry, and corn grown using conventional, organic, and sustainable agricultural practices. *Journal of Agricultural Food Chemistry* 2003; 51: 1237–1241.

9. Worthington, V. Nutritional quality of organic versus conventional fruits, vegetables, and grains. *Journal of Alternative and Complementary Medicine* 2001; 7: 161–173.

10. Curl, C. L.; Fenske, R. A.; and Elgethun, K. Organophosphorus pesticide exposure of urban and suburban preschool children with organic and conventional diets. *Environmental Health Perspectives* 2003; 111 (3): 377–382.

Chapter 4. Supplement Savvy

1. Beaudin, A. E., and Stover, P. J. Insights into metabolic mechanisms underlying folate-responsive neural tube defects: a minireview. *Birth Defects Research. Part A Clinical and Molecular Teratolology* 2009; 85 (4): 274–284.

2. Julvez, J.; Fortuny, J.; Mendez, M.; et al. Maternal use of folic acid supplements during pregnancy and four-year-old neurodevelopment in a population-based birth cohort. *Paediatric Perinatal Epidemiology* 2009; 23 (3): 199–206.

3. Roza, S. J.; van Batenburg-Eddes, T.; Steegers, E.A.P.; et al. Maternal folic acid supplements use in early pregnancy and child behavioural problems: The Generation R Study. *British Journal of Nutrition* 2010; 103 (3): 445–452.

4. Nelen, W. L.; Blom, H. J.; Steegers, E. A.; et al. Homocysteine and folate

levels as risk factors for recurrent early pregnancy loss. *Obstetrics & Gynecology* 2000; 95: 519–524.

5. Elkin, A. C., and Higham, J. Folic acid supplements are more effective than increased dietary folate intake in elevating serum folate levels. *British Journal of Obstetrics & Gynaecology* 2000; 107: 285–259.

6. Heiss, C. J.; Shaw, S. E.; and Carothers, L. Association of calcium intake and adiposity in postmenopausal women. *Journal of the American College of Nutrition* 2008; 27 (2): 260–266.

7. Kulie, T.; Groff, A.; Redmer, J.; et al. Vitamin D: an evidence-based review. *Journal of the American Board of Family Medicine* 2009 (November–December); 22 (6): 698–706.

8. Binkley, N.; Novotny, R.; Krueger, D.; et al. Low vitamin D status despite abundant sun exposure. *Journal of Clinical Endocrinology Metabolism* 2007; 92 (6): 2130–2135.

9. Holmes, V. A.; Barnes, M. S.; Alexander, H. D.; et al. Vitamin D deficiency and insufficiency in pregnant women: a longitudinal study. *British Journal of Nutrition* 2009 (September); 102 (6): 876–881.

10. Haugen, M.; Brantsaeter, A. L.; Trogstad, L.; et al. Vitamin D supplementation and reduced risk of preeclampsia in nulliparous women. *Epidemiology* 2009 (September); 20 (5): 720–726.

11. Kremer, R.; Campbell, P. P.; Reinhardt, T.; et al. Vitamin D status and its relationship to body fat, final height, and peak bone mass in young women. *Journal of Clinical Endocrinology Metabolism* 2009; 94 (1): 67–73.

Chapter 5. Fitting in Exercise

1. Marshall, S. J.; Levy, S. S.; Tudor-Locke, C. E.; et al. Translating physical activity recommendations into a pedometer-based step goal: 3000 steps in 30 minutes. *American Journal of Preventive Medicine* 2009; 36 (5): 410–415.

2. Maughan, R. J. Impact of mild dehydration on wellness and on exercise performance. *European Journal of Clinical Nutrition* 2003; 57 (suppl 2): S19–S23.

3. Cheuvront, S. N.; Carter, R.; and Sawka, M. N. Fluid balance and endurance exercise performance. *Current Sports Medical Report* 2003; 2 (4): 202–208.

4. Hinton, P. S.; Giordano, C.; Brownlie, T.; et al. Iron supplementation improves endurance after training in iron-depleted, nonanemic women. *Journal of Applied Physiology* 2000; 88: 1103–1111.

5. Spodaryk, K.; Czekaj, J.; and Sowa, W. Relationship among reduced level of stored iron and dietary iron in trained women. *Physiology Research* 1996; 45:

393–397.

6. Malczewska, J.; Raczynski, G.; and, Stupnicki, R. Iron status in female endurance athletes and in nonathletes. *International Journal of Sports Nutrition & Exercise Metabolism* 2000; 10: 260–276.

7. Friedmann, B.; Weller, E.; Mairbaurl, H.; et al. Effects of iron repletion on blood volume and performance capacity in young athletes. *Medical Science Sports Exercise* 2001; 33: 741–746.

8. Hinton, P. S.; Giordano, C.; Brownlie, T.; et al. Iron supplementation improves endurance after training in iron-depleted, nonanemic women. *Journal of Applied Physiology* 2000; 88: 1103–1111.

9. Matheson, G. O. Sports: Hazardous to your health? *Physician Sportsmedicine* 2003; 31 (10):2.

10. Lohmander, L. S.; Ostenberg, A.; Englund, M.; et al. High prevalence of knee osteoarthritis, pain, and functional limitations in female soccer players twelve years after anterior cruciate ligament injury. *Arthritis & Rheumatism* 2004; (10): 3145–3152.

11. Krumbach, C. J.; Ellis, D. R.; and Driskell, J. A. A report of vitamin and mineral supplement use among university athletes in a division I institution. *International Journal of Sports Nutrition* 1999; 9: 416–425.

12. Sen, C. K. Antioxidants in exercise nutrition. *Sports Medicine* 2001; 31 (13): 891–908.

13. Varma, S. D.; Hegde, K.; and Henein, M. Oxidative damage to mouse lens in culture. Protective effect of pyruvate. *Biochimica et Biophysica Acta* 2003; 1621 (3): 246–252.

14. Ivy, J. L. Effect of pyruvate and dihydroxyacetone on metabolism and aerobic endurance capacity. *Medical Science & Sports Exercise* 1998; 30 (6): 837–843.

15. Nieman, D. C.; Henson, D. A.; Gross, S. J.; et al. Quercetin reduces illness but not immune perturbations after intensive exercise. *Medical Science & Sports Exercise* 2007; 39: 1561–1569.

16. Karlic, H., and Lohninger, A. Supplementation of L-carnitine in athletes: does it make sense? *Nutrition* 2004; 20 (7–8): 709–715.

17. Connolly, D. A.; McHugh, M. P.; Padilla-Zakour, O. I.; et al. Efficacy of a tart cherry juice blend in preventing the symptoms of muscle damage. *British Journal of Sports Medicine* 2006; 40 (8): 679–683.

18. Widrig, R.; Suter, A.; Saller, R.; et al. Choosing between NSAID and arnica for topical treatment of hand osteoarthritis in a randomised, double-blind study. *Rheumatology International* 2007; 27 (6): 585–591.

Chapter 6. Rediscovering Beauty Basics

1. Stahl, W., and Sies, H. Carotenoids and flavonoids contribute to nutritional protection against skin damage from sunlight. *Molecular Biotechnology* 2007; 37 (1): 26–30.

2. Jeon, H. Y.; Kim, J. K.; Kim, W. G.; et al. Effects of oral epigallocatechin gallate supplementation on the minimal erythema dose and UV-induced skin damage. *Skin Pharmacology & Physiology* 2009; 22 (3): 137–141.

3. Barel, A.; Calomme, M.; Timchenko, A.; et al. Effect of oral intake of choline-stabilized orthosilicic acid on skin, nails and hair in women with photodamaged skin. *Archives of Dermatological Research* 2005; 297 (4): 147–153.

4. Afaq, F., and Mukhtar H. Botanical antioxidants in the prevention of photo-carcinogenesis and photoaging. *Experimental Dermatology* 2006; 15 (9): 678–684.

5. Farris, P. K. Topical vitamin C: a useful agent for treating photoaging and other dermatologic conditions. *Dermatological Surgery* 2005; 31 (7 Pt 2): 814–817.

6. Beitner, H. Randomized, placebo-controlled, double blind study on the clinical efficacy of a cream containing 5% alpha-lipoic acid related to photoageing of facial skin. *British Journal of Dermatology* 2003; 149 (4): 841–849.

7. Blatt, T.; Mundt, C.; Mummert, C.; et al. Modulation of oxidative stresses in human aging skin. *Gerontology & Geriatrics* 1999; 32 (2): 83–88.

8. De Spirt, S.; Stahl, W.; Tronnier, H.; et al. Intervention with flaxseed and borage oil supplements modulates skin condition in women. *British Journal of Nutrition* 2009; 101 (3):440–445.

9. Wickett, R. R.; Kossmann, E.; Barel, A.; et al. Effect of oral intake of choline-stabilized orthosilicic acid on hair tensile strength and morphology in women with fine hair. *Archives of Dermatological Research* 2007; 299 (10): 499–505.

10. Zschocke, I.; Radtke, M. A.; Cummerow, R.; et al. A pilot study on the efficacy of silicium gel on the thickness of hair in healthy women with thin hair. *Kosmetische Medizin* 2007; 6: 23–27

11. Jones, C.; Woods, K.; Whittle, G.; et al. Sugar, drinks, deprivation and dental caries in 14-year-old children in the north west of England in 1995. *Community Dental Health* 1999; 16 (2): 68–71.

12. Linke, H. A., and LeGeros, R. Z. Black tea extract and dental caries formation in hamsters. *International Journal of Food Science & Nutrition* 2003; 54 (1): 89–95.

13. Pai, M. R.; Acharya, L. D.; and Udupa, N. Evaluation of antiplaque activity of *Azadirachta indica* leaf extract gel—a 6-week clinical study. *Journal of Ethnopharmacology* 2004; 90: 99–103.

14. Edgar, W. M. Sugar substitutes, chewing gum and dental caries—a review. *British Dental Journal* 1998; 184: 29–32.

15. Nase, L.; Hatakka, K.; Savilahti, E.; et al. Effect of long-term consumption of a probiotic bacterium, *Lactobacillus rhamnosus* GG, in milk on dental caries and caries risk in children. *Caries Research* 2001; 35: 412–420.

16. Moore, C.; Addy, M.; and Moran, J. Toothpaste detergents: a potential source of oral soft tissue damage? *International Journal of Dental Hygiene* 2008; 6 (3): 193–198.

17. Kibayashi, M.; Tanaka, M.; Nishida, N.; et al. Longitudinal study of the association between smoking as a periodontitis risk and salivary biomarkers related to periodontitis. *Journal of Periodontics* 2007; 78 (5): 859–867.

Chapter 7. Reconnecting with Passion

1. Lake, Polan M. Abstract appearing in *Journal of Women's Health & Gender-Based Medicine* 2001; 10: 401.

2. Estrada-Reyes, R.; Ortiz-Lopez, P.; Gutierrez-Ortiz, J.; et al. *Turnera diffusa* wild (Turneraceae) recovers sexual behavior in sexually exhausted males. *Journal of Ethnopharmacology* 2001; 123: 423–429.

3. Oh, K. J.; Chae, M. J.; Lee, H. S.; et al. Effects of Korean red ginseng on sexual arousal in menopausal women: placebo-controlled, double-blind crossover clinical study. *Journal of Sexual Medicine* 2010; 7: 1469–1477.

4. Shin, B. C.; Lee, M. S.; Yang, E. J.; et al. Maca (*L. meyenii*) for improving sexual function: a systematic review. *BMC Complementary & Alternative Medicine* 2010; 10: 44.

5. Waynberg, J., and Brewer, S. Effects of Herbal vX on libido and sexual activity in premenopausal and postmenopausal women. *Advanced Therapies* 2000; 17: 255–262.

Chapter 8. Fighting Fatigue

1. Lopez-Garcia, E.; van Dam, R. M.; Li, T. Y.; et al. The relationship of coffee consumption with mortality. *Annals of Internal Medicine* 2008; 148 (12): 904–914.

2. Ganmaa, D.; Willett, W. C.; Li, T. Y.; et al. Coffee, tea, caffeine and risk of breast cancer: a 22-year follow-up. *International Journal of Cancer* 2008; 122 (9): 2071–2076.

3. Roth, T.; Krystal, A. D.; and Lieberman, J. A. Long-term issues in the treatment of sleep disorders. *CNS Spectrums* 2007; 12 (7 Suppl 10): 1–14.

4. Nathan, P. J.; Lu, K.; Gray, M.; et al. The neuropharmacology of L-theanine (N-ethyl-L-glutamine): a possible neuroprotective and cognitive enhancing agent. *Journal of Herbal Pharmacology* 2006; 6 (2): 21–30.

5. L-Tryptophan. Monograph. *Alternative Medicine Review* 2006 ;11 (1): 52–56.

6. Dimpfel, W., and Suter, A. Sleep improving effects of a single dose administration of a valerian/hops fluid extract. *European Journal of Medical Research* 2008; 13: 1–5.

7. Puri, B. K. The use of eicosapentaenoic acid in the treatment of chronic fatigue syndrome. *Prostaglandins, Leukotrienes and Essential Fatty Acids* 2004; 70: 399–401.

8. Monograph. L-carnitine. *Alternative Medicine Review* 2005; 10 (1): 42–50.

9. Lee, K. A.; Zaffke, M. E.; and Baratte-Beebe, K. Restless legs syndrome and sleep disturbance during pregnancy: the role of folate and iron. *Journal of Women's Health & Gender-Based Medicine* 2001; 10: 335–341.

Chapter 9. Stress and Sanity

1. Tsang, H. W.; Fung, K. M.; Chan, A. S.; et al. Effect of a qigong exercise programme on elderly with depression. *International Journal of Geriatric Psychology* 2006; 21: 890–897.

2. Levant, B. N-3 (omega-3) Fatty acids in postpartum depression: implications for prevention and treatment. *Depression Research & Treatment* 2011; 2011: 467349.

3. Norman, E.; Sherburn, M.; Osborne, R. H.; et al. An exercise and education program improves well-being of new mothers: a randomized controlled trial. *Physical Therapy* 2010; 90 (3): 348–355.

4. Coppen, A., and Bailey, J. Enhancement of the antidepressant action of fluoxetine by folic acid: a randomized, placebo controlled trial. *Journal of Affective Disorders* 2000; 60: 121–130.

5. Gastpar, M.; Singer, A.; and Zeller, K. Efficacy and tolerability of hypericum extract STW3 in long-term treatment with a once-daily dosage in comparison with sertraline. *Pharmacopsychology* 2005; 38: 78–86.

6. Bell, I.; Edman, J.; Morrow, F.; et al. B complex vitamin patterns in geriatric and young adult inpatients with major depression. *Journal of the American Geriatric Society* 1991; 39: 252–257.

7. Benton, D. Selenium intake, mood and other aspects of psychological functioning. *Nutritional Neuroscience* 2002 (December); 5 (6): 363–374.

8. Paluska, S. A., and Schwenk, T. L. Physical activity and mental health: current concepts. *Sports Medicine* 2000; 29: 167–180.

9. Ross, B. M. Omega-3 polyunsaturated fatty acids and anxiety disorders. *Prostaglandins, Leukotrienes, and Essential Fatty Acids* 2009; 81 (5–6): 309–312.

10. Hamazaki, K.; Itomura, M.; Huan, M.; et al. Effect of omega-3 fatty acid-containing phospholipids on blood catecholamine concentrations in healthy volunteers: a randomized, placebo-controlled, double-blind trial. *Nutrition* 2005; 21 (6): 705–710.

11. Panossian, A.; Wikman, G.; and Sarris, J. Rosenroot (*Rhodiola rosea*): traditional use, chemical composition, pharmacology and clinical efficacy. *Phytomedicine* 2010; 17 (7): 481–493.

12. Silveri, M. M.; Dikan, J.; Ross, A. J.; et al. Citicoline enhances frontal lobe bioenergetics as measured by phosphorus magnetic resonance spectroscopy. *NMR Biomedicine* 2008; 21 (10): 1066–1075.

13. Monograph. Phosphatidylserine. *Alternative Medicine Review* 2008; 13 (3): 245247.

14. Kennedy, D. O.; Haskell, C. F.; Mauri, P. L.; et al. Acute cognitive effects of standardised *Ginkgo biloba* extract complexed with phosphatidylserine. *Human Psychopharmacology* 2007; 22 (4): 199–210.

15. Ryan, J.; Croft, K.; Mori, T.; et al. An examination of the effects of the antioxidant Pycnogenol on cognitive performance, serum lipid profile, endocrinological and oxidative stress biomarkers in an elderly population. *Journal of Psychopharmacology* 2008; 22 (5): 553–562.

16. Valikovics, A. Investigation of the effect of vinpocetine on cerebral blood flow and cognitive functions. *Ideggyógyászati Szemle* 2007; 60 (7–8): 301–310.

17. Neilson, H. K.; Friedenreich, C. M.; Brockton, N. T.; et al. Physical activity and postmenopausal breast cancer: proposed biologic mechanisms and areas for future research. *Cancer Epidemiology & Biomarkers Prevention* 2009 (January); 18 (1): 11–27.

Chapter 10. After-Baby Health Concerns

1. Fogarty, A.; Lewis, S. A.; Scrivener, S. L.; et al. Corticosteroid sparing effects of vitamin C and magnesium in asthma: a randomised trial. *Respiratory Medicine* 2006; 100 (1): 174–179.

2. Monograph. *Petasites hybridus*. *Alternative Medicine Review* 2001; 6 (2): 207–209.

3. Danesch, U. C. *Petasites hybridus* (Butterbur root) extract in the treatment of asthma—an open trial. *Alternative Medicine Review* 2004; 9 (1): 54–62.

4. Gagnier, J. J.; van Tulder, M. W.; Berman, B.; et al. Herbal medicine for low back pain: a Cochrane review. *Spine* 2007; 32 (1): 82–92.

5. Cade, J. E.; Burley, V. J.; Greenwood, D. C.; et al. Dietary fibre and risk of breast cancer in the UK Women's Cohort Study. *International Journal of Epidemiology* 2007; 36 (2): 431–438.

6. Slavin, J. L. Position of the American Dietetic Association: health implications of dietary fiber. *Journal of the American Dietetic Association* 2008; 108 (10): 1716–1731.

7. Shrubsole, M. J.; Lu, W.; Chen, Z.; et al. Drinking green tea modestly reduces breast cancer risk. *Journal of Nutrition* 2009; 139 (2): 310–316.

8. Dugoua, J. J.; Seely, D.; Perri, D.; et al. Safety and efficacy of chastetree (Vitex agnus-castus) during pregnancy and lactation. *Canadian Journal of Clinical Pharmacology* 2008; 15 (1): e74–e79.

9. Hemila, H., and Douglas, R. M. Vitamin C and acute respiratory infections. *International Journal of Tubercular Lung Disease* 1999; 3: 756–761.

10. Sasazuki, S.; Sasaki, S.; Tsubono, Y.; et al. Effect of vitamin C on common cold: randomized controlled trial. *European Journal of Clinical Nutrition* 2006; 60 (1): 9–17.

11. Prasad, A. S.; Fitzgerald, J. T.; Bao, B.; et al. Duration of symptoms and plasma cytokine levels in patients with the common cold treated with zinc acetate. A randomized, double-blind, placebo-controlled trial. *Annals of Internal Medicine* 2000; 133: 245–252.

12. Oliff, H. S., and Blumenthal, M. Andrographis-eleuthero combination for upper respiratory tract infections in colds and flus. *HerbalGram* 2005; 66: 26–27.

13. Bergmann, J.; Luft, B.; Boehmann, S.; et al. The efficacy of the complex medication Phyto-Hypophyson L in female hormone-related sterility. A randomized, placebo-controlled clinical double-blind study. *Forsch Komplementarmed Klass Naturheilkd* 2000; 7: 190–199.

14. Marzari, R.; Mazzanti, P.; Cazzola, P.; et al. Perennial allergic rhinitis: prevention of the acute episodes with Thymomodulin. *Minerva Medica* 1987; 78: 1675–1681.

15. Diener, H. C.; Pfaffenrath, V.; Schnitker, J.; et al. Efficacy and safety of 6.25 mg t.i.d. feverfew CO_2-extract (MIG-99) in migraine prevention—a randomized, double-blind, multicentre, placebo-controlled study. *Cephalalgia* 2005; 25 (11): 1031–1041.

16. Woolhouse, M. Migraine and tension headache. *Australian Family Physician* 2005; 34 (8): 647–650.

17. Sandor, P. S.; Di Clemente, L.; Coppola, G.; et al. Efficacy of coenzyme Q$_{10}$ in migraine prophylaxis: a randomized controlled trial. *Neurology* 2005; 64 (4): 713–715.

18. Dominguez-Munoz, J. E.; Iglesias-Garcia, J.; Inglesias-Rey, M.; et al. Effect of the administration schedule on the therapeutic efficacy of oral pancreatic enzyme supplements in patients with exocrine pancreatic insufficiency: a randomized, three-way crossover study. *Alimentary Pharmacological Therapies* 2005; 21 (8): 993–1000.

19. Pirotta, M. Irritable bowel syndrome. *Australian Family Physician* 2009; 38 (12): 966–968.

20. Merat, S.; Khalili, S.; Mostajabi, P.; et al. The effect of enteric-coated, delayed-release peppermint oil on irritable bowel syndrome. *Digestive Disease Science* 2010; 55 (5): 1385–1390.

21. Jass, J., and Reid, G. Effect of cranberry drink on bacterial adhesion *in vitro* and vaginal microbiota in healthy females. *Canadian Journal of Urology* 2009 December; 16 (6): 4901–4907.

22. Bailey, D. T.; Dalton, C.; Daugherty, J.; et al. Can a concentrated cranberry extract prevent recurrent urinary tract infections in women? A pilot study. *Phytomedicine* 2007; 14 (4): 237–241.

23. McMurdo, M. E.; Argo, I.; Phillips, G.; et al. Cranberry or trimethoprim for the prevention of recurrent urinary tract infections? A randomized controlled trial in older women. *Journal of Antimicrobial Chemotherapy* 2009; 63 (2): 389–395.

24. Reid, G., and Bruce, A. W. Probiotics to prevent urinary tract infections: the rationale and evidence. *World Journal of Urology* 2006; 24 (1): 28–32.

25. Hilton, E.; Isenberg, H. D.; Alperstein, P.; et al. Ingestion of yogurt containing Lactobacillus acidophilus as prophylaxis for candidal vaginitis. *Annals of Internal Medicine* 1992 (March) 1; 116 (5): 353–357.

Appendix. Herb and Dietary Supplement Safety

1. Low Dog, T. The use of botanicals during pregnancy and lactation. *Alternative Therapies in Health & Medicine* 2009; 15 (1): 54–58.

2. Aston, J. L.; Lodolce, A. E.; and Shapiro, N. L. Interaction between warfarin and cranberry juice. *Pharmacotherapy* 2006; 26 (9): 1314–1319.

3. Dugoua, J. J.; Seely, D.; Perri, D.; et al. Safety and efficacy of cranberry (*Vac-*

cinium macrocarpon) during pregnancy and lactation. *Canadian Journal of Clinical Pharmacology* 2008; 15 (1): e80–e86.

4. Low Dog, T. The use of botanicals during pregnancy and lactation. *Alternative Therapies in Health & Medicine* 2009; 15 (1): 54–58.

5. Dugoua, J. J.; Mills, E.; Perri, D.; et al. Safety and efficacy of ginkgo (*Ginkgo biloba*) during pregnancy and lactation. *Canadian Journal of Clinical Pharmacology* 2006; 13 (3): e277–e284.

6. Low Dog, T. The use of botanicals during pregnancy and lactation. *Alternative Therapies in Health & Medicine* 2009; 15 (1): 54–58.

7. Low Dog, T. The use of botanicals during pregnancy and lactation. *Alternative Therapies in Health & Medicine* 2009; 15 (1): 54–58.

8. Kendall-Tackett, K. Long-chain omega-3 fatty acids and women's mental health in the perinatal period and beyond. *Journal of Midwifery & Women's Health* 2010; 55 (6): 561–567.

9. Dugoua, J. J.; Mills, E.; Perri, D.; et al. Safety and efficacy of St. John's wort (hypericum) during pregnancy and lactation. *Canadian Journal of Clinical Pharmacology* 2006 Fall;13 (3): e268–e276.

10. Dugoua, J. J.; Seely, D.; Perri, D.; et al. Safety and efficacy of chastetree (*Vitex agnus-castus*) during pregnancy and lactation. *Canadian Journal of Clinical Pharmacology* 2008; 15 (1): e74–e79.

Index

About the Author

Victoria Dolby Toews, MPH

In school, Victoria Dolby Toews studied health and received her master of public health degree, but she always knew she wanted to write as well. Her solution? She became a health journalist. For the past two decades she's been reading highly scientific literature, learning about hot-off-the-press medical discoveries, and incorporating all the best parts into her writing. She's the author of several books, including *The Green Tea Book*. She has written hundreds of magazine articles about achieving wellness through natural medicine and dietary supplements. She lives in the Pacific Northwest with her husband, son, and daughter.